Contemporary Diagnosis and Management of Otitis Media

Russell W. Steele, MD

Professor and Vice Chairman of Pediatrics,
Division Head, Infectious Diseases,

and

Dana L. Suskind-Liu, MD

Assistant Professor of Otolaryngology—
Head and Neck Surgery

Louisiana State University
School of Medicine
and Children's Hospital
New Orleans, LA

First Edition

Published by
Handbooks in Health Care Co.
Newtown, Pennsylvania, USA

This book has been prepared and is presented as a service to the medical community. The information provided reflects the knowledge, experience, and personal opinions of Russell W. Steele, MD, Professor and Vice Chairman of Pediatrics, Division Head, Infectious Diseases, and Dana L. Suskind-Liu, MD, Assistant Professor of Otolaryngology, LSU School of Medicine, Children's Hospital, New Orleans, LA.

This book is not intended to replace or to be used as a substitute for the complete prescribing information prepared by each manufacturer for each drug. Because of possible variations in drug indications, in dosage information, in newly described toxicities, in drug/drug interactions, and in other items of importance, reference to such complete prescribing information is definitely recommended before any of the drugs discussed are used or prescribed.

International Standard Book Number: 1-884065-45-7

Library of Congress Catalog Card Number: 98-74011

Contemporary Diagnosis and Management of Otitis Media®. Copyright© 2000 by Handbooks in Health Care Co., a Division of AMM Co., Inc. All rights reserved. Printed in the United States of America. No part of this book may be used or reproduced in any manner whatsoever without written permission, except in the case of brief quotations embodied in critical articles and reviews. For information, write Handbooks in Health Care, 3 Terry Drive, Suite 201, Newtown, Pennsylvania 18940, (215) 860-9600. Web site: www.HHCbooks.com.

Table of Contents

Introduction

Pediatricians spend an estimated 30% of their time managing otitis media, second only to well-child care in clinical responsibilities. Early and aggressive intervention is essential for the child's comfort, as well as for prevention of severe suppurative complications of otitis media such as mastoiditis and meningitis. Also, prevention of persistent conductive hearing loss, which delays speech development and cognitive function, is equally important. A highly organized yet individualized approach to therapy and follow-up is therefore essential for each pediatric patient and for the efficient operation of an entire office practice.

Many researchers speculate that the increase in the prevalence of otitis media results from more children in out-of-home child care. An estimated 12 million children attend these facilities more than 20 hours a week, and another 5 million spend at least some time there. Clearly, children attending nonresidential centers, particularly facilities that serve 13 or more children in a partial-day or full-day program, have more episodes of acute otitis media, and their first occurrence occurs at an earlier age compared with children who stay at home. Concern is also growing over the potential overdiagnosis of otitis media and concomitant overuse of antibiotics. This concern can be partially addressed by reference sources such as this, which offer practitioners detailed information on the diagnosis and management of this common outpatient pediatric infection.

The purpose of this handbook is to provide a comprehensive resource to physicians who care for patients with otitis media, to minimize both short-term and long-term sequelae. This is a challenging time for a handbook, because the selection of antibiotics for common outpatient infections is undergoing significant change, primarily because antimicrobial susceptibilities of common pathogens are rapidly changing.

This handbook reviews all aspects of middle ear disease, from both the medical and surgical standpoints, and emphasizes the responsibilities of primary care physicians in caring for these patients. Resources include all available literature, but we emphasize guideline recommendations generated by the American Academy of Pediatrics, the American Academy of Family Physicians, and the American Academy of Otolaryngology—Head and Neck Surgery, as well as other authoritative groups. We do so because these recommendations are more likely to influence the approach to treating middle ear disease. We also carefully review aspects normally addressed by otolaryngologists so that primary care physicians can better understand the surgical management of patients who do not respond to the usual medical interventions.

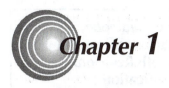

Chapter 1

Definitions and Epidemiology

Interpretation of published clinical literature that addresses management of inflammatory conditions of the middle ear often is difficult, primarily because definitions of disease have varied. Publications designed to evaluate the antibiotic treatment of uncomplicated acute otitis media are particularly difficult. The Medicode International Classification of Diseases, 9th Revision, Clinical Modification (ICD-9) codes for otitis media use wording that is much different from current medical terminology (Table 1). Any survey that uses these limited codes for tracking physician practices obviously is combining a number of pathologic processes. Determination of the incidence and management of otitis media with effusion is particularly difficult because it cannot be clearly identified by any ICD-9 code.

Definitions

The definitions listed below are those suggested in numerous guideline recommendations published by the American Academy of Pediatrics and, more recently, the Infectious Diseases Society of America, which established firm definitions of acute otitis media for implementation in investigative studies.[1] For purposes of simplification, abbreviations for common middle ear diseases will be used (Table 2) and every attempt is made to separate these various forms of ear disease in analyzing published literature.

Table 1: Otitis Media: Medicode International Classification of Diseases, 9th Revision, Clinical Modification

Diagnosis	ICD-9
Bullous myringitis	384.01
Otalgia	388.70
Otitis media, acute, purulent	382.00
Otitis media, chronic, purulent	382.3
Otitis media, rupture	382.01
Otitis serous, acute	381.01
Otitis serous, chronic	381.10
Otorrhea	388.60
Perforation of eardrum	384.20

Table 2: Common Abbreviations

OM—otitis media (all forms)

AOM—acute otitis media

OME—otitis media with effusion

CSOM—chronic suppurative otitis media

Otitis Media (OM): The general wording for infection or inflammatory changes of the middle ear. Unfortunately, this term includes acute and chronic processes, with or without the presence of middle ear effusion. Therefore, conditions such as myringitis, middle ear serous effusion, and even simple retraction of the tympanic membrane all may be described in literature with the inclusive term *otitis media.*

Table 3: IDSA-FDA Guidelines for Diagnosis of AOM: Signs and Symptoms That Define Middle Ear Disease[1]

Specific signs	*Nonspecific signs*
• Otalgia	• Fever
• Otorrhea	• Irritability
• Hearing loss	• Lethargy
• Vertigo	• Anorexia
	• Vomiting
	• Diarrhea

Acute Otitis Media (AOM): A diagnosis of AOM requires the presence of middle ear effusion along with the rapid onset of clinical signs and symptoms, most commonly fever, pain, irritability, anorexia, or vomiting (Table 3).[1] This definition separates AOM from otitis media with effusion (OME), which is not associated with symptoms, and from chronic suppurative otitis media (CSOM), which is a persistent inflammatory process with a perforated tympanic membrane and draining exudate for more than 6 weeks. Effusion must be identified by direct visualization of the tympanic membrane using a pneumatic otoscope, or by aural acoustic immittance measurement, to fully evaluate movement of the membrane (Table 4). Chapter 5 includes a complete outline of diagnostic methods.

Otitis Media with Effusion (OME): Fluid in the middle ear without signs or symptoms of ear infection is the definition of OME established by the Otitis Media Guideline Panel,[2] reviewed in depth in Chapter 11. Because all cases of AOM begin with middle ear effusion, once acute signs

**Table 4:   IDSA-FDA Guidelines
for Diagnosis of AOM:
Methods for Documenting
Middle Ear Effusion[1]**

- Pneumatic otoscopy
  - Decreased mobility
  - Air fluid level/bubbles
- Tympanometry
- Acoustic reflectometry

and symptoms resolve, these patients would be classified on reexamination as having OME until fluid is no longer present. Persistence of middle ear effusion requires management interventions, as indicated in Chapter 11. OME may also represent one aspect of upper respiratory allergy or accumulation of serous fluid from obstruction of the eustachian tubes. This most frequently results from upper respiratory viral infections, which cause mild inflammation of the mucosal lining in eustachian tubes and in other posterior pharyngeal and middle ear structures.

Chronic Suppurative Otitis Media (CSOM): Persistent infection of the middle ear and mastoid air cells accompanied by otorrhea through a perforated tympanic membrane for at least 6 weeks. Such chronic disease without cholesteatoma should be distinguished from CSOM with cholesteatoma, because management is quite different. The latter is primarily a surgical disease, while CSOM without cholesteatoma can be managed medically, as described in Chapter 12. In addition to otorrhea, patients usually experience ear pain and variable hearing loss. CSOM rarely responds to first-line antimicrobial therapy that is effective in the treatment of AOM. The chronic

Table 5: Risk Factors for Recurrent Acute Otitis Media (AOM)

Factors that can be influenced

- Parental smoking
- Total bottle feeding
- Anatomic defects (cleft palate)
- Immune deficiency
- Inadequate medical care
- Poor sanitation

Factors that may potentially be influenced

- Large-group day care
- Poverty
- Crowded living conditions

Factors that cannot be influenced

- Male gender
- Ethnic groups (American Indian, Eskimos)
- First episode at early age
- First episode caused by *Streptococcus pneumoniae*
- Sibling or parental history of recurrent AOM
- Season (winter, fall)

infection may lead to irreversible damage to ear ossicles, with resulting conductive and sensorineural hearing loss.

Epidemiology

AOM is by far the most common infectious disease encountered in clinical practice, occurring primarily in

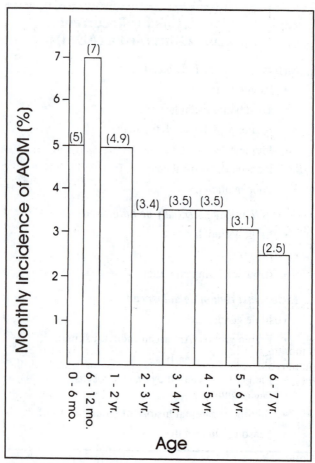

Figure 1: *Age-specific incidence of otitis media, combining data from four independent studies.*[3-6]

young children, but occasionally in adolescents and adults. An understanding of the epidemiologic features of OM offers limited but important information to guide preventive measures and to anticipate recurrent or progressively severe disease (Table 5). Because virtually all children experience at least one episode of acute infection, most recommendations for controlling OM are universal. On the other hand, recognition of certain high-risk groups allows for identification of children who might need special attention.

The natural history of disease suggests that although infection usually occurs without obvious antecedent factors, many episodes are preceded by viral upper respiratory illness in children with an anatomic predisposition to eustachian tube dysfunction.[3-7] This is particularly true for patients with a history of recurrent or chronic ear infection. More simply, certain children seem to develop AOM whenever they have colds. Parents are quick to recognize this pattern, particularly when another child in the family has demonstrated the same predisposition.

Two thirds of infants have at least one episode before their first birthday, and virtually all have an episode by age 5.[8-11] A number of epidemiologic studies have emphasized that OM is a disease of the latter part of infancy and of early childhood.[12-15] A typical survey demonstrated an increasing incidence of OM, from 29% during the first 6 months of life to a maximum of 42% in infants 6 to 12 months old, and then a decreasing incidence through childhood[12] (Figure 1).

Total visits and proportions of pediatrician visits by children in Boston for middle ear disease between 1975 and 1982 were determined.[12] These data were extrapolated nationally, yielding 24 million visits a year in the United States during this period. Using similar survey methods, cases in Boston now translate to more than 20 million office visits a year for initial management of acute middle ear disease, and at least an equal number of encounters for follow-up assessment and additional treatment of failures, a figure confirmed by independent studies conducted at the Centers for Disease Control and Prevention (Table 6).[16]

Table 6:	Office Visits for Otitis Media, United States, 1975-2000[11]	
Year	**No. of Visits (millions)**	
1975	9.9	
1980	14.1	
1985	18.3	
1990	24.5	
1997	29.6	
2000 (projected)	34.8	

Investigations that examined these data from another perspective determined that, on average, children are treated with antibiotics for OM for 41 to 45 days in each of the first 2 years of life.[17] Also, a very recent study conducted in private practice settings in Atlanta, which examined the impact of current management on individual children, found that children received an average of 0.4 to 9.0 courses of antibiotics a year.[18]

The incidence of OM in the United States can also be calculated by reviewing overall oral antibiotic use and use specifically related to the management of ear infections. Data from the National Ambulatory Medical Care Survey (NAMCS) project a total of 128 million antibiotic prescriptions in 1998 for both children and adults, an increase of 40 million prescriptions over the previous 2 decades.[16] Shortly after 1990, OM became the most common diagnosis requiring antibiotics; other diagnoses, in order of decreasing frequency, were upper respiratory tract infections, bronchitis, pharyngitis, sinusitis, and acne. An independent 1996 study by the Institute of Medicine looking at diagnosis-specific use of antibiotics revealed that approximately 24 million prescriptions for antibiotic suspensions were written for the treatment of OM.[19] This study concluded that 30 million prescriptions would be written in 1998, and estimated that figure to climb to 40 million for OM by 2000, almost twice the number filled in 1980. These estimates, based on current and projected antibiotic use, are very close to those calculated in the clinical survey studies reviewed above.

Critical review and interpretation of the survey data rapidly reveal one of the major shortcomings of otitis media literature: distinction between the various forms of middle ear disease. In diagnosis-related survey studies, office visits for suspected ear infections may be for treatment of acute infection, follow-up to document resolution of uncomplicated cases, changes in antimicrobial therapy for treatment failures, or evaluation of chronic cases. This shortcoming therefore casts some doubt on the incidence figures determined by either survey or antibiotic-use data.

Although the incidence of uncomplicated AOM has risen, sequelae of both acute and chronic disease have decreased considerably. In 1939, Bellevue Hospital in New York City reported that 27% of all pediatric admissions were for suppurative consequences of middle ear infection, primarily mastoiditis and intracranial complications.[20] Mastoidectomy scars were common in individuals who were born in the 1920s and 1930s, before the availability of effective antimicrobial agents and aggressive early medical management of middle ear infection. The introduction of sulfonamides in 1935 and penicillin in 1941 greatly changed the natural history of OM. In contrast to the relatively recent medical approaches to disease, surgical management dates back to 1736, when the first successful operation for mastoiditis was performed. Thus, for more than 200 years, OM was considered a surgical disease that was treated with myringotomy when needed, or with aggressive surgical intervention for more serious suppurative sequelae. Otherwise, disease resolved spon-

Table 7: Long-Term Morbidity of Otitis Media

- Middle ear effusion
- Conductive hearing loss
- Decreased perception of language
- Impaired development of speech and language
- Lower scores on tests of cognitive abilities
- Poor performance in school

taneously, resulted in perforation of the tympanic membrane and eventual resolution of infection, or progressed to a more unfortunate outcome.

In addition to alleviating acute discomfort and preventing extension of infection, aggressive early management of AOM offers the best potential for reversing both acute and chronic auditory dysfunction, a quality-of-life issue for young children (Table 7). This hearing loss may delay cognitive development, particularly normal speech patterns[21] (Chapter 3). Adults would be unlikely to tolerate this degree of hearing loss for more than a few days, yet clinicians continue to debate the need for aggressive management in young children. The overall interpretation of the day-to-day importance of hearing loss in children influences various management options. If the auditory changes are considered inconsequential, delayed therapy or even no therapy at all could be considered for AOM.[22] Most primary care physicians have concluded that hearing loss is indeed an important medical event, and that persistence of middle ear fluid warrants aggressive management to its resolution.

Viral Respiratory Infections

The incidence of AOM clearly increases during outbreaks of viral infection, particularly those caused by res-

Table 8: Viral URI and Otitis Media[21]

Virus	Otitis Media (%)
-	7
RSV	33
Adenovirus	28
RSV and adenovirus	73
Influenza A and B	28
Parainfluenza	15
Rhinovirus	10

piratory syncytial virus (RSV), but is also well documented with rhinovirus, influenza, parainfluenza, and adenovirus disease[3,6] (Table 8). Because these epidemics generally occur during the winter and early spring, the similar seasonal distribution of ear infection can be attributed to antecedent viral initiating events. Inflammation produced by these viral infections progresses to eustachian tube obstruction, serous fluid accumulation, and subsequent growth of colonizing bacteria within the middle ear cavity. During the progression of these events, responsible viruses can be cultured from the throat, posterior nasopharynx, and the middle ear itself. This pattern has been documented in more than 25% of AOM cases in children younger than 3 years old.[5] The most convincing studies isolated viruses or viral antigens from middle ear fluids.[3,4] With newer virus identification techniques, more than 1 in 6 cases of AOM have been associated with middle ear viral colonization, most in conjunction with bacterial pathogens. Twice this number of documented bacterial ear infections (ie, 2 in 6) occur in association with nasopharyngeal viral disease. During RSV outbreaks, this association is much greater: RSV can be isolated from the upper respiratory tract or middle ear in 64% of all bacterial AOM cases.[6] RSV as a predisposing factor to AOM is even more apparent in studies that examined the natural history of RSV in infants. Two thirds of all RSV-infected children develop AOM during the course of infection, a sufficient incidence to support routine antimicrobial therapy once RSV is identified in children with symptomatic pulmonary disease.

When viral and bacterial pathogens coexist, treatment with antibiotics results in slower resolution and a higher frequency of both microbiologic and clinical failures, compared with disease produced by bacteria alone. Recent data suggest that this may result from decreased penetration of antibiotics into the middle ear attributable to the presence of viral pathogens and viral-induced inflammation.[4]

In addition to common respiratory viral agents, AOM may follow a number of other systemic viral illnesses, most prominently measles, Epstein-Barr virus-related infectious mononucleosis, and decades ago, smallpox. The mechanism by which these viruses predispose to secondary bacterial infection in the middle ear is presumed to be similar to that for respiratory viruses.

Seasonal Distribution

AOM occurs most often in the winter months, with an increased incidence in the early spring and fall. The prevalence of asymptomatic middle ear effusion also follows a similar seasonal distribution in studies that examined children for middle ear fluid at various times of the year. For example, in a study of children less than 5 years old, middle ear effusion occurred in none during the summer and in less than 10% in the early fall, but in 25% of all children in the winter months.[6] Other studies have shown that effusions persist longer in the winter than in the summer.

The seasonal pattern for OM more closely follows that of upper respiratory tract pathogens, rather than that of asthma and other allergic diatheses caused by environmental agents such as pollens or grasses. These observations have cast doubt on the need to routinely consider an allergy evaluation for children with recurrent otitis or persistent middle ear effusion.

Day-Care Center Attendance

After viral upper respiratory infections, the next most prominent risk factor for recurrent OM and persistence of middle ear effusion is attendance at large day-care centers, an epidemiologic factor with some options for intervention. Children rarely can be totally managed at home because so many mothers with preschool-aged children work outside the home for economic reasons or personal satisfaction. Other parents use these facilities to allow personal time for social activities. The availability of care outside large centers should be explored for children who are otitis media-prone (see Chapter 9).

Numerous studies have compared the incidence of OM for children cared for at home to that for children in group day care. The incidence is higher by 25% or more for those in group day care, and the difference is even more striking for predisposition to recurrent infection. The need for ventilating-tube placement and myringotomy was also 7-fold higher for children in group day care.[23]

The risk in day-care centers is attributable to the constant and close exposure to other young children who may harbor respiratory pathogens and transmit them to their susceptible playmates. Epidemics of viral disease are quite common in this setting, transmitted not only by coughing or sneezing, but also by contamination of fomites. Observations of toddlers in day-care environments have shown that these young children place some object in their mouth more than once a minute. At this age, children are quite sharing with one another, and of course are too young to understand the risks of such behavior.

Respiratory pathogens such as RSV and rhinovirus may remain viable for hours or even days on fomites such as toys, particularly if they remain moist from secretions. The sharing of these toys by children greatly increases the potential for colonization with viral pathogens. Therefore, washing and drying of toys at least daily is recommended as routine policy in child-care facilities.

Allergy

Allergy is thought to play only a minor role because the incidence of OM does not increase during the summer and fall, when inhalant allergens and resultant allergic diatheses are more common. However, allergy may be important for some children, particularly those with prominent upper respiratory symptoms during allergic exacerbations.

All of the evidence linking allergy to OM is indirect. No investigations have clearly demonstrated a convincing pathogenetic mechanism. In addition, conclusions have conflicted in published studies that were designed to examine epidemiologic patterns or markers for allergy in children with OM. This lack of consensus likely results from inadequate research design. Many studies showing increased positivity of allergy skin testing or radioallergosorbent test (RAST) in patients with recurrent OM are inherently biased because they were usually conducted in allergy referral settings.[24]

Various local respiratory markers for allergy have been shown to be positive in patients with AOM. Examples include nasal eosinophilia, immunoglobulin E (IgE) in middle ear fluid, and mast cells in middle ear mucosa.[25] However, these findings do not confirm cause and effect because they are nonspecific, and because other environmental factors may still have had a greater influence in predisposing to acute disease. More importantly, studies have been unable to delineate the sequence of pathologic events to determine whether infection itself might account for some of these local changes before the appearance of allergic manifestations.

Anatomic Abnormalities

Propensity to ear infection is clearly increased in children with craniofacial malformations,[26-27] pointing out once again that OM is not purely an infectious disease. The best example of this association is children with cleft palate, in whom recurrent infection is so common that most experts recommend prophylactic antibiotics and ventilating tubes.[27] At least some disease in these children results from milk or other liquids causing inflammation of the eustachian tubes. Another example of anatomic predisposition is children with Down syndrome, who have eustachian dysfunction as a result of craniofacial abnormalities and an alteration in the position of the bony eustachian tube. Researchers also hypothesize that the lower incidence of disease in African-American children is related to differences in the morphology of the eustachian tube and surrounding cranial structures.[26]

Genetic Factors

The well-appreciated predilection to recurrent AOM among children in certain families implies a genetic predisposition, most likely based on anatomic variations. The main factor also could be immunologic, but this has been carefully studied, and proof is lacking. The anatomy of the cranial base and eustachian tubes was carefully studied in American Indian Apache children and Eskimos, two groups with an extremely high incidence of OM. These groups had morphologic variations conducive to the development of middle ear infections.[28] This study remains the most convincing and quoted publication that addresses the potential for genetic influences.

Age and Sex

Disease in children peaks between 6 and 18 months of age, when anatomic structures are small and viral diseases are frequent. Like most infections, incidence is somewhat higher in boys. This results from the subtle immune enhancement provided by genes carried on X chromosomes.

Prematurity and low birth weight have not been shown to predispose children to ear infection, with the single exception of one study of Australian children whose birth weight was less than 1,500 g.[29] These premature infants had a significantly higher incidence of both OM and short-term hearing loss.

Race

African-American children usually have a significantly lower incidence of middle ear infection and hearing impairment than do white children in the United States.[26,30] The two explanations for this difference are each supported only by limited data. One explanation is anatomic differences based on genetic influences. The other suggests an overall lower number of medical visits for African-American children usually included in clinical research studies.

Conclusion

Epidemiologic patterns favor antecedent viral infections, along with an anatomic predisposition in children, as the most important factors for subsequent chronic or recurrent ear infections. Day-care center attendance, particularly in large-group facilities, greatly increases the likelihood of disease, because young children are likely to transmit viral infections to others in such settings.

References

1.   Chow AW, Hall CB, Klein JO, et al: Evaluation of new anti-infective drugs for the treatment of respiratory tract infections. Infectious Diseases Society of America and the Food and Drug Administration. *Clin Infect Dis* 1992;15:S62-S88.

2.   The Otitis Media Guideline Panel: Managing otitis media with effusion in young children. American Academy of Pediatrics. *Pediatrics* 1994;94:766-773.

3.   Pitkaranta A, Virolainen A, Jero J, et al: Detection of rhinovirus, respiratory syncytial virus, and coronavirus infections in acute

otitis media by reverse transcriptase polymerase chain reaction. *Pediatrics* 1998;102:291-295.

4.   Canafax DM, Yuan Z, Chonmaitree T, et al: Amoxicillin middle ear fluid penetration and pharmacokinetics in children with acute otitis media. *Pediatr Infect Dis J* 1998;17:149-156.

5.   Ruuskanen O, Arola M, Heikkinen T, et al: Viruses in acute otitis media: increasing evidence for clinical significance. *Pediatr Infect Dis J* 1991;10:425-427.

6.   Henderson FW, Collier AM, Sanyal MA, et al: A longitudinal study of respiratory viruses and bacteria in the etiology of acute otitis media with effusion. *N Engl J Med* 1982;306:1377-1383.

7.   Giebink GS, Mills EL, Huff JS, et al: The microbiology of serous and mucoid otitis media. *Pediatrics* 1979;63:915-919.

8.   Steele RW: Management of otitis media. *Infect Med* 1998;15: 174-178, 203.

9.   Klein JO: Otitis media. *Clin Infect Dis* 1994;19:823-833.

10. Chartrand SA, Pong A: Acute otitis media in the 1990s: the impact of antibiotic resistance. *Pediatr Ann* 1998;27:86-95.

11. Berman S: Otitis media in children. *N Engl J Med* 1995; 332:1560-1565.

12. Teele DW, Klein JO, Rosner B: Epidemiology of otitis media during the first seven years of life in children in greater Boston: a prospective, cohort study. *J Infect Dis* 1989;160:83-94.

13. Howie VM: Natural history of otitis media. *Ann Otol Rhinol Laryngol* 1975;84:67-72.

14. Wright PF, McConnell KB, Thompson JM, et al: A longitudinal study of the detection of otitis media in the first two years of life. *Int J Pediatr Otorhinolaryngol* 1985;10:245-252.

15. Kero P, Piekkala P: Factors affecting the occurrence of acute otitis media during the first year of life. *Acta Paediatr Scand* 1987;76:618-623.

16. McCaig LF, Hughes JM: Trends in antimicrobial drug prescribing among office-based physicians in the United States. *JAMA* 1995;273:214-219.

17. Dowell SF, Marcy MS, Phillips WR, et al: Otitis media—principles of judicious use of antimicrobial agents. *Pediatrics* 1998; 101:165-171.

18. Dowell SF, Schwartz B: Resistant pneumococci: protecting patients through judicious use of antibiotics. *Am Fam Physician* 1997;55:1647-1654.

19. Schappert SM: Office visits for otitis media: United States, 1975-90. From: Vital and Health Statistics of the Centers for Disease Control/National Center for Health Statistics, 1992, pp 1-18.

20. Bakwin H, Jacobinzer H: Prevention of purulent otitis media in infants. *J Pediatr* 1939;14:730-736.

21. Roberts JE, Burchinal MR, Zeisel SA, et al: Otitis media, the caregiving environment, and language and cognitive outcomes at 2 years. *Pediatrics* 1998;102:346-354.

22. Bauchner H, Philipp B: Reducing inappropriate oral antibiotic use: a prescription for change. *Pediatrics* 1998;102:142-145.

23. Wald ER, Dashefsky B, Byers C, et al: Frequency and severity of infections in day care. *J Pediatr* 1988;112:540-546.

24. Mogi G: Immunologic and allergic aspects of otitis media. In: Lim DJ, Bluestone CD, Klein JO, et al, eds. *Recent Advances in Otitis Media With Effusion.* Burlington, Ontario, Decker Periodicals, 1993, pp 145-151.

25. Bernstein JM: The role of IgE-mediated hypersensitivity in the development of otitis media with effusion. *Otolaryngol Clin North Am* 1992;25:197-211.

26. Doyle WJ: *A Function-Anatomic Description of Eustachian Tube Vector Relations in Four Ethnic Populations—An Osteologic Study* (dissertation). University of Pittsburgh, 1977.

27. Paradise JL, Bluestone CD: Early treatment of the universal otitis media of infants with cleft palate. *Pediatrics* 1974;53:48-54.

28. Beery QC, Doyle WJ, Cantekin EI, et al: Eustachian tube function in an American Indian population. *Ann Otol Rhinol Laryngol Suppl* 1980;89:28-33.

29. Kitchen WH, Ford GW, Doyle LW, et al: Health and hospital readmissions of very-low-birth-weight and normal-birth-weight children. *Am J Dis Child* 1990;144:213-218.

30. Marchant CD, Shurin PA, Turczyk VA, et al: Course and outcome of otitis media in early infancy: a prospective study. *J Pediatr* 1984;104:826-831.

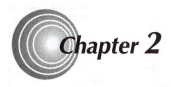

Chapter 2

Anatomy, Physiology, and Pathophysiology

The anatomy and maturation of the middle ear system, specifically the eustachian tube (ET), are intimately related to the incidence and pathophysiology of acute otitis media (AOM) in the pediatric population. The network of contiguous structures that make up the middle ear system includes the nose, nasopharynx, ET, middle ear, and mastoid (Figure 1). Pathologic changes in this network—such as infection, inflammation or obstruction involving any part of the system—may manifest as middle ear pathology.

Anatomy and Physiology

The middle ear cleft is an aerated, irregularly shaped space bound laterally by the tympanic membrane, superiorly by the tegmen (the separation between the middle cranial fossa and middle ear), medially by the labyrinthine wall (inner ear), and inferiorly by the jugular bulb (Figure 2). The carotid artery and eustachian tube are located anteriorly. The middle ear cleft is covered by ciliated respiratory epithelium that is contiguous throughout the entire middle ear system. The ossicular chain (malleus, incus, and stapes) and the facial nerve are located within the middle ear cleft. The ossicular chain provides the conductive aspect of sound transmission (Figure 3). This sound conduction is sensitive to pathology within the middle ear; a clear middle ear equalized to atmospheric

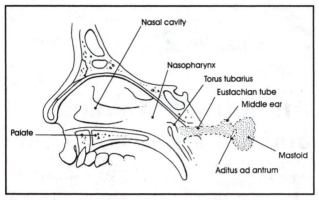

Figure 1: The middle ear system. Adapted from Bluestone CD, Klein JD, eds: Otitis Media in Infants and Children, 2nd ed. Philadelphia, WB Saunders, 1995.

pressure is the most efficient and effective environment for sound transmission.

The tympanic membrane is a window into the middle ear cleft and system. It is composed of three layers: an outer squamous, a middle fibrous, and an inner mucosal layer. The thin and translucent tympanic membrane allows for indirect visualization into the middle ear, and also acts as an indicator of recurrent infections. Tympanic membrane perforations often heal in only two layers, without the middle fibrous layer, resulting in a monomer.

The mastoid cavity is posterior to the middle ear space, and is composed of, and partitioned by, pneumatized air cells. The antrum is the connection between the middle ear and mastoid cavity, just posterior to the epitympanum. Some researchers believe the mastoid acts as a pressure equalizer in ET dysfunction and negative middle ear pressure. Mastoid pneumatization is progressive: the infant mastoid is small and underdeveloped, and becomes larger and pneumatized with age. Frequent bouts of OM often result in an underdeveloped, underpneumatized mastoid.

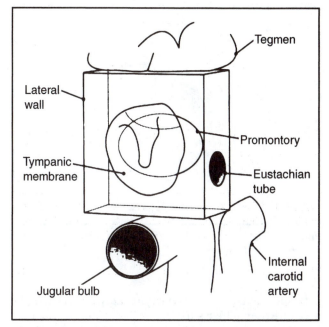

Figure 2: *Boundaries of the middle ear cleft. Adapted from Bluestone CD, Klein JD, eds:* Otitis Media in Infants and Children, *2nd ed. Philadelphia, WB Saunders, 1995.*

The mastoid tip is the palpable inferior portion of the mastoid, attached to the sternocleidomastoid in adults. In infants and children less than 2 years old, the mastoid tip is not yet developed, leaving the facial nerve, as it exits the mastoid, exposed and vulnerable during surgery.

The nasopharynx is posterior to the nasal cavity; the soft palate forms the floor, and the base of skull forms the roof. The ET drains into the lateral nasopharynx, and is demarcated by a prominence of soft tissue over cartilage, the torus tubarius. Posterior to the torus tubarius is a deep, mucosa-lined pocket, Rosenmüller's fossa, and anteriorly is the orifice to the ET. The adenoid pad, lo-

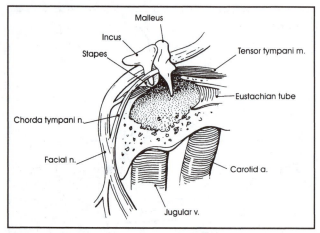

Figure 3: *The ossicular chain (malleus, incus, and stapes) and the facial nerve are located within the middle ear cleft.*

cated in the posterior nasopharynx, may extend into the area of Rosenmüller's fossa.

The status of the middle ear is closely tied to the function and dysfunction of the ET. The ET connects the middle ear with the nasopharynx, and is divided into an anterior fibrocartilaginous portion (2/3) and a posterior osseous portion (1/3). Its narrowest portion is the isthmus, approximately 1 mm wide and 2 mm high. The isthmus represents the junction between the fibrocartilaginous and osseous portions. Only the osseous portion is continually open; the fibrocartilaginous portion is closed at rest and opens during specific actions, such as Valsalva's maneuver and swallowing. The ET has a ciliated mucosal lining that is contiguous with the middle ear and nasopharyngeal mucosal lining. This lining is sensitive to the status of the mucosa throughout the sinonasal tract and middle ear system. Thus, an upper respiratory tract infection that results in sinonasal edema may also result in ET edema.

Table 1: Eustachian Tube Functions

- Middle ear ventilation
- Middle ear drainage
- Middle ear protection

The lymphoid tissue within the ET is referred to as Gerlach's tonsils.

Four muscles are intimately related to the ET: the tensor tympani, the levator veli palatini, the salpingopharyngeus, and the tensor veli palatini. The tensor veli palatini is most associated with ET dilation, and results in inferolateral displacement of the fibrocartilaginous ET. Its importance in ET function is demonstrated most prominently in cleft palate patients, whose difficulty with recurrent middle ear infections stems from the dysfunction of the tensor tympani.

Physiology of the Eustachian Tube

The ET has three main physiologic functions: (1) ventilation of the middle ear and equilibration with atmospheric pressure; (2) drainage and clearance of middle ear secretions into the nasopharynx; and (3) protection of the middle ear from sound and nasopharyngeal secretions (Table 1).

Middle ear ventilation is the most important function of the ET, and its dysfunction is often the primary cause of OM. The ET is closed in the resting state, and opens with actions such as yawning and Valsalva's maneuver. This allows for equilibration with atmospheric pressure in the middle ear, a state that is optimal for hearing. The tensor veli palatini is the only ET muscle involved in active dilation. With ET dysfunction and resultant impairment of middle ear ventilation, negative pressure develops in the middle ear. The normal middle ear resting

Table 2: Differences Between the Infant and Adult Eustachian Tube

- Less angle (10 degrees vs 45 degrees)
- Shorter length/equal width
- Less efficient tensor veli palatini
- Overall less effective ET function

pressure in most children is between 0 and -175 mm H_2O. Under normal conditions, the rate of gas absorption from the middle ear is about 1 mL every 24 hours. Negative pressure in the middle ear may lead to a transudative serous effusion or nasopharyngeal bacterial reflux into the middle ear, leading to OM. Reflux of nasopharyngeal secretions may occur because of the pressure gradient between the positive pressure of the nasopharynx and the negative middle ear pressure. Prolonged negative middle ear pressure eventually leads to an atrophic, retracted tympanic membrane, much as an overstretched balloon loses its elasticity. Structural changes occur within the tympanic membrane, converting the trilayer membrane into a bilayer membrane with inflammation rather than fibrous tissue intervening.

The ET also protects the middle ear from nasopharyngeal secretions and bacteria. This may be visualized as a flask: the long narrow neck is the ET, and its chamber is the mastoid. The capillarity within the ET and the positive pressure in the chamber prevent secretions within the ET from entering the mastoid. In infants and children, the ET is shorter, but is as wide as that in adults. This leads to a decreased surface tension and capillarity and a higher incidence of reflux from the nasopharynx into the middle ear, resulting in compromised protection. In addition,

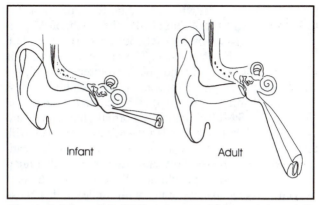

Figure 4: *The adult ET lies at a 45-degree angle, while the infant ET is positioned at a 0- to 10-degree angle.*

negative middle ear pressure and the common supine position of infants add to the risk of 'reflux otitis media.'

Finally, the ET drains the middle ear via a combination of factors, including mucociliary transport of the ET and middle ear, the pumping action that results from the opening and closing of the ET, and the surface tension factors of the ET. Studies have demonstrated surface tension-lowering substances in the ET, similar to surfactant. Negative pressure in the middle ear results in secretions being 'locked' in the middle ear and unable to drain through the ET. When a myringotomy tube is placed or when the tympanic membrane spontaneously ruptures, the 'suction' is broken and the effusion can drain.

A number of anatomic and thus functional differences between the infant and adult ET secondarily affect the middle ear status of infants (Table 2). In contrast to the adult size of the middle ear at birth, the newborn ET is between 17 and 18 mm, compared to the 31 to 38 mm of the adult ET. This shorter ET may predispose the middle ear to increased nasopharyngeal reflux. The adult ET lies at a 45-degree angle, while the infant ET is positioned at a 0- to 10-degree angle (Figure 4). The height of the pharyngeal orifice is approximately 50% of that of the adult, while the width is adult size. The tensor veli palatini is less efficient in infants and young children. Overall, the ET function of even otologically normal children is less effective than in adults. Studies have demonstrated that more than 33% of otologically normal children are unable to equilibrate 100 mm H_2O of negative pressure with swallowing, compared with only 5% of adults who cannot complete this task. Further studies indicate that function improves with age: children between 3 and 6 years old are less able to equilibrate their middle ear than those between 7 and 12 years. This is consistent with the decrease in incidence of OM with an increase in age.

Pathogenesis

Numerous interrelated factors are involved in the pathogenesis of OM, including ET dysfunction (functional and mechanical), allergy and immunology status, active infection, and environmental exposure. ET dysfunction is regarded as the central factor in the pathophysiology of OM. The associated causes most often primarily affect ET function, resulting in OM. The mechanisms addressed below result in disruption of one or more of the ET functions: ventilation, protection, and clearance (Table 1).

ET obstruction and abnormal patency both result in ET dysfunction, leading to OM. Tubal obstruction is by far the most common dysfunction, and may stem from either failure to dilate (functional) or anatomic obstruction (mechanical). Functional ET impairment occurs in the pediatric population because of failure of the active opening mechanism (eg, an inefficient tensor veli palatini) or of an overly compliant, collapsible cartilaginous tube (eg, an immature infant ET) (Figure 5a). Anatomic obstruction occurs because of noninherent factors such as environmental allergies, resulting in peritubal inflammation

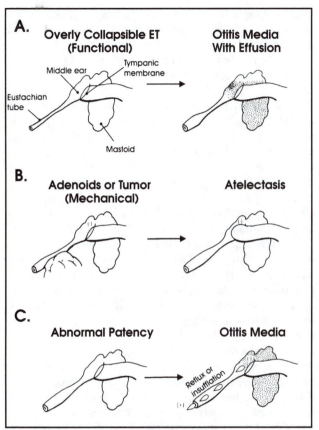

Figure 5: *(5a, 5b, 5c) Impairments of eustachian tube function. Adapted from Bluestone CD, Klein JD, eds: Otitis Media in Infants and Children, 2nd ed. Philadelphia, WB Saunders, 1995.*

or extrinsic obstruction, resulting from adenoid hypertrophy, nasotracheal intubation, or malignancy (Figure 5b).

An abnormally patent or patulous ET is an unusual cause of OM in children, and is most common with significant weight loss (Figure 5c). In this situation, the ET is either open even at rest, or has a decreased resistance and thus decreased opening pressure. Some American Indians have been shown to have a decreased tubal resistance and increased incidence of nasopharyngeal reflux and OM.

Researchers have long theorized that allergy is a factor in OM, but little scientific literature supports this in the pediatric population. Clinicians have hypothesized that pathogenesis is related to mucosal edema of the ET, to reflux of infected nasopharyngeal secretions into the middle ear, or to nasal congestion resulting in equalization dysfunction of the ET. In support of these hypotheses, many allergic patients have concomitant OM as well as mast cells and an elevated IgE in their middle ear mucosa.

The postulated role of adenoid hypertrophy as a cause of OM is multifactorial. First, lymphoid hypertrophy may cause direct mechanical obstruction of the nasopharyngeal orifice of the ET. It may also result in obstruction of the posterior choanae with swallowing, resulting in increased nasopharyngeal pressure and bacterial reflux into the ET. Finally, a chronically infected adenoid pad may increase the risk of bacteria-laden nasopharyngeal secretion reflux into the middle ear. These theories remain controversial, and some have already been contradicted in the scientific literature. Overall, studies have demonstrated the efficacy of adenoidectomy for recurrent OM. Interestingly, the effect of adenoidectomy on OM does not depend on the size of the adenoid pad.

Cleft palate infants have been shown to have an incidence of middle ear effusion (MEE) of more than 94%. This is caused by an ineffective tensor veli palatini and resultant functional ET obstruction. The tensor veli palatini arises from the skull base and inserts into the lateral palate. In cleft patients, the tensor veli palatini is dehiscent because of the loss of the muscles' midline insertion. Cleft palate repair decreases the incidence of OM, although it does not eliminate it. Children with submucous clefts and even bifid uvulae have been shown to have an increased incidence of OM, which is also probably caused by functional obstruction.

Diseases that affect ciliary function also affect mucociliary flow, and thus drainage of the middle ear. Ciliary dysfunction may be genetic or acquired from infection. Children with defective ciliary function classically present with the triad of recurrent sinusitis, pneumonia, and OM. Viral infections and smoke exposure may cause transient ciliary dysfunction.

Selected Readings

Anatomy. In: Bluestone CD, Klein JO, eds. *Otitis Media in Infants and Children*. Philadelphia, WB Saunders, 1995, pp 5-16.

Bluestone CD: Anatomy and physiology of the eustachian tube. In: Bailey BJ, ed. *Head and Neck Surgery—Otolaryngology*. Philadelphia, JB Lippincott, 1993, pp 1473-1482.

Physiology, pathophysiology and pathogenesis. In: Bluestone CD, Klein JO, eds. *Otitis Media in Infants and Children*. Philadelphia, WB Saunders, 1995, pp 5-16.

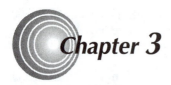

Chapter 3

Persistent Middle Ear Effusion and Cognitive Development

After an episode of acute otitis media (AOM), middle ear effusion (MEE), by definition initially present in all children, persists for a variable period of time[1] (Figure 1), creating a mild to moderate fluctuating hearing loss. Accumulated fluid remains sufficient to distort the tympanic membrane for 3 to 4 weeks, but 20% of children have a clinically significant effusion for 8 weeks, and 10% for 12 weeks. This information is useful for determining the best time for routine follow-up of patients with AOM and for implementation of appropriate interventions. Other patients with otitis media with effusion (OME) may be identified during routine examination or screening with no history suggestive of earlier AOM (Table 1). In these children, MEE may persist even longer[2] (Figure 1).

When fluid persists, discrimination and processing of speech is impaired, and the child may miss or confuse educational information relevant to language and cognitive skills. Parents, caregivers, and educators may interpret this as the child's lack of interest, and decrease the interactions necessary for optimal intellectual achievement.[3] Of course, it is difficult to determine which variable in this sequence contributes most to the resulting developmental delay.

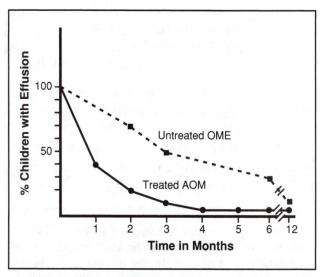

Figure 1: *Persistence of middle ear effusion after a single episode of AOM or after identification of OME.[1,2]*

Medical interventions that have been shown to result in more rapid resolution of MEE include early antimicrobial therapy for AOM, a repeat course of antibiotics for persistent effusion, oral corticosteroids, and ventilating (tympanostomy or pressure equalization) tubes.[4] Other popular therapies that do not appear to be effective are nasal and oral decongestants, antihistamines, and various combinations of these agents.

All of these options were critically evaluated in the clinical practice guidelines for OME in young children, published in 1994 by the Otitis Media Guideline Panel.[5] The algorithm for management of these patients is provided in Chapter 11, Figure 1. This panel of health-care providers in various subspecialties developed the guidelines after comprehensively analyzing the research literature and scientific knowledge of the development, diag-

Table 1: OME and Hearing Loss
(≥25 dB Hearing Level)
During the First 2 Years of Life[3]

Age in months	Percentage (%) of Time ± Standard Deviation			
	Bilateral OME	Unilateral OME	Total OME	Hearing Loss
6-14	68 ± 29	15 ± 15	83 ± 25	55 ± 31
15-24	31 ± 34	14 ± 13	46 ± 34	33 ± 34
6-24	49 ± 30	14 ± 10	63 ± 26	44 ± 29

nosis, and treatment of OME in children 1 to 3 years old with no craniofacial or neurologic abnormalities or sensory deficits. The panel restricted its analysis to the earlier results of randomized, controlled clinical trials. In doing so, combination therapy with an antibiotic plus a corticosteroid for persistent effusion, compared with an antibiotic alone, was interpreted as approaching but not fulfilling criteria for clinical significance (25% vs 21% clearance of effusions). On the other hand, longer follow-up did show significant differences. Using the same endpoint, either an antibiotic alone or the combination were clearly superior to placebo. The panel subsequently did not recommend an antibiotic plus a corticosteroid. The value of corticosteroids as adjunctive therapy remains debatable.

If corticosteroid therapy is chosen, a regimen of oral prednisone 0.5 to 1.0 mg/kg/d q 24 h for 7 days, along with an antibiotic effective against likely pathogens given as a prolonged course (21 days), appears best supported by published clinical trials.[4]

Nasal aerosolized corticosteroids have not been shown to benefit children with MEE,[6] although clinical trials have been limited.

Bilateral Versus Unilateral MEE

Unilateral hearing loss attributable to persistent OME is generally assumed to have no clinical significance. Virtually all studies examining the possibility that OME is associated with cognitive impairment have therefore only evaluated children with bilateral fluid. Interestingly, of all children who have OME lasting longer than 12 weeks, 68% have bilateral fluid and hearing loss, while only 15% have unilateral retention of fluid with resulting hearing impairment. Approximately 17% have either bilateral or unilateral MEE unassociated with an elevation in the threshold for speech reception.[3] Thus, for children with OME and hearing loss, bilateral effusions are more than 4 times as common as unilateral effusions. This suggests a difference in the natural history of bilateral versus unilateral AOM.

The assumption that unilateral hearing loss is not associated with impaired cognitive development has been called into question in studies of children with unilateral sensorineural (rather than conductive) deficits, in that test scores for auditory-dependent skills have been consistently abnormal.[7] Similar data are not available for unilateral conductive losses, but many experts have concluded that consequences should be identical. Virtually all studies examining OME and auditory function have identified children with unilateral OME with abnormally elevated hearing thresholds for speech, when sounds are presented simultaneously to both ears.[3]

OME and Delayed Cognitive Development

The effusions that persist after AOM almost always produce a conductive hearing loss and occasionally a sensorineural deficit. The severity of hearing loss (Table 2) appears to be a major determinant of resultant cognitive delay, although data have not absolutely defined the relationships among OME, the severity of auditory dysfunction, and intellectual progression. In contrast, sensorineu-

Table 2: Classification of Hearing Loss (HL) Based on Threshold for Speech Reception

Speech Threshold Decibels (dB)	Interpretation
0-20 dB	normal
25-40 dB	mild HL
40-55 dB	moderate HL
55-70 dB	moderately severe HL
70-90 dB	severe HL
>90 dB	profound HL

ral abnormalities have clearly been shown to delay language development, and a relationship with severity of hearing impairment has been established.

The conductive hearing loss attributable to MEE as a cause of reduced language and learning skills has not been fully established, primarily because a number of potential confounding variables have not been adequately analyzed. These include the child's environment, age of onset for middle ear disease, and severity and duration of hearing impairment.

Studies Supporting a Relationship

Investigations of OM sequela published 16 to 31 years ago are still often quoted, but are generally retrospective and involve a relatively small number of study patients[8-14] (Table 3). Some focus on populations known to have a very high predisposition to recurrent AOM, such as Eskimo children.[9] In such populations, the natural history of MEE may be different from that observed in other populations. The general format of these studies was to test

Table 3: Otitis Media With Effusion and Observed Cognitive Development Association

Study	Conclusion	Comment
Holm, Kunze 1969[8]	Language skills delayed	16 children with chronic OM before 2 years; 16 controls
Kaplan, et al 1973[9]	Lower test scores in reading, math, and language at age 10 years	Eskimo children 0 to 4 years of age; recurrent otorrhea
Lewis 1976[10]	Reduced speech and language development	Australian aboriginal children, 7 to 9 years old; 14 with effusion and hearing deficit; 18 controls
Needleman 1977[11]	Delayed speech skills	Recurrent OM; 20 children 3 to 8 years old; 20 controls
Sak, Ruben 1981[12]	Lower verbal IQ; reduced spelling proficiency	Persistent OM; testing at 8 to 11 years of age; sibling controls
Friel-Patti 1982[13]	Language delay	Premature infants with early-onset AOM
Teele et al 1984[14]	Lower speech and language test scores	Prospective monitoring of 205 children, birth to 3 years

language skills in children with a history of chronic OM defined in various ways, and to compare these test results with those of control populations. Typical of the earlier investigations was one that included a sample size of only 16 children and 16 controls. It concluded that those language skills that require normal speech reception were delayed, while skills relying on visual or motor processing were normal.[8]

The best investigations focusing on MEE and development of speech and language were undertaken by the Greater Boston Otitis Media Study Group, which began enrollment of patients for prospective evaluation in the mid-1970s.[14] The group's first assessment of data studied 205 3-year-old children, each of whom were examined frequently from birth. Both the number of episodes of AOM and persistence of OME were monitored. Standardized tests of speech and language were administered to all children at age 3. Those who had prolonged periods of OME had lower speech and language test scores than did those without long intervals of middle ear disease. The correlation was greater in children from higher socioeconomic families. This study, as well as most others, indicates that recurrent OME at an early age, usually defined as less than 18 months, is critical in differences in subsequent testing of cognitive skills.

Continued investigations by the Boston group included an equal number of children from these same geographic and socioeconomic backgrounds followed from birth to age 7 years. Intellectual ability was tested with the Wisc-R performance IQ test.[15] Results are summarized in Table 4. A reduction in IQ scores of 7% to 8% occurred in children who had MEE for more than 130 days. Results were similar for both verbal and performance testing. In these studies, confounding variables were carefully controlled so that differences attributable to time spent with MEE during the first 3 years of life could be examined as an independent variable.

Table 4:	Cognitive Ability at Age 7 Years by Estimated Days With Middle Ear Effusion (MEE) During the First 3 Years of Life[15]		

| | Estimated Days with MEE | | |
IQ Test	<30	30-129	>130
Full scale	113.1	107.5	105.4
Verbal	111.5	106.5	105.8
Performance	112.2	108.3	104.1

Sak and Ruben monitored a relatively large population of infants and young children using sibling controls for study cases with recurrent OM.[12] In this investigation, patients were selected based on a history of persistent OM before 5 years of age, along with a sibling whose history was negative for similar pathology. Testing of these children was similar to that of the Boston group, and likewise revealed a lower verbal IQ and lower scores on other measures of cognitive development.

Studies Not Supporting a Relationship

Similar to the clinical studies by the Boston group, investigators in Nashville, Tenn followed 210 normal, healthy children from birth longitudinally through the first 2 years of life with frequent pneumatic otoscopy and tympanometry[16] (Table 5). These children were from mostly lower socioeconomic status families, and included 130 white and 80 black children. All episodes of AOM were treated with oral antibiotics, and children were seen 3 weeks after each acute episode and at 1- to 2-month intervals until resolution of MEE. At 2 years of age, the children underwent hearing and cognitive evaluations.

Table 5:   Otitis Media With Effusion and Cognitive Development Association Not Observed

Study	Conclusion	Comment
Wright PF et al 1988[16]	Normal speech and language development	Prospective monitoring of 210 children, birth to 2 years
Roberts JE et al 1995[17]	Normal language and cognitive measures	61 black infants, tested at age 1 year
Feagans L et al 1994[18]	Normal language development	Upper middle class, two parent, dual-earner families
Roberts JE et al 1998[3]	Minor effect on cognitive skills	86 African-American low-income families

Speech and language development were appraised by a comprehensive battery of tests. None of the otitis-related variables influenced speech, language, or developmental tests used in this study. Hearing evaluation was repeated at 3 to 4 years of age and, by this time, the association between hearing loss and prior OM was no longer evident. By this age, all children had normal hearing when they were retested. This study concluded that, although recurrent OM induces a temporary decrease in hearing sensitivity evident at 2 years of age, it is not associated with a delay in language acquisition or cognitive development, and the hearing loss resolves by 3 to 4 years of age. A similar study in rural North Carolina, which examined cognitive and verbal ability in 3 1/2- to 5-year-old children with various durations of OME, likewise showed no correlation between verbal ability and the duration of effusion.[17] Both of these studies examined children of lower socioeconomic status, which may be an important cofactor that influences overall cognitive development for children with hearing impairment.

Parenting as a Central Factor

A recent prospective serial assessment of children during the first 2 years of life indicated a correlation between hearing loss and reduced cognitive function.[3] The study examined 86 African-American infants, 6 to 12 months old, who attended group child care centers in suburban and rural North Carolina. They came predominantly from single-parent, low-income families. The mean IQ of the primary guardian was 87.2. In analyzing all variables, however, the central factor resulting in intellectual delay appeared to be a poor caregiving environment. Correction for this variable negated a direct relationship between OME and language and intellectual skills. Thus, children in lower-quality homes and poor parenting environments have more OME with hearing loss in addition to lower scores on cognitive skills testing, which may or may not primarily relate to decreased auditory function. In contrast to this study, other investigations have not shown a difference in the interaction patterns of mothers whose children have persistent OME, compared with mothers of children without chronic middle ear disease.[18-20] The differences in these studies may be attributable to the population groups studied; the publication from North Carolina[3] included only African-American children attending community-based child-care programs. Such children are known to have an unusually high prevalence of OME. It is difficult to compare data and conclusions from this study to those that have focused predominantly on middle- and high-income families. The latter environments likely offer a more consistent and responsive interactive style from parents and from providers in relatively expensive child-care programs. Considerable data support these variables as important in facilitating children's language development.

If an association exists between the caregiving environment and intellectual development, an indirect link to persistent MEE may also exist. In lower-quality homes and child-care environments, duration of breast-feeding is shorter; smoking, crowding, exposure to more children, and bottle propping are increased; access to medical care is decreased; and hygiene is poorer. All of these factors independently predispose to recurrent OM. Some parents may not interact well with their children, and this deficiency is accentuated when the child has delayed language skills. Such a conclusion is based on the premise that a great deal of education in young children comes from parental involvement and the parents' interest in their child's intellectual achievements. Parenting skill is a confounding variable that cannot be quantitated. Moreover, the relative influence of each variable (ie, otitis media, persistent middle ear effusion, hearing loss, and the caregiving environment) remains speculative.

References

1.   Teele DW, Klein JO, Rosner BA: Epidemiology of otitis media in children. *Ann Otol Rhinol Laryngol Suppl* 1980;89:5-6.

2.   Zielhuis GA, Straatman H, Rach GH, et al: Analysis and presentation of data on the natural course of otitis media with effusion in children. *Int J Epidemiol* 1990;19:1037-1044.

3.   Roberts JE, Burchinal MR, Zeisel SA, et al: Otitis media, the caregiving environment, and language and cognitive outcomes at 2 years. *Pediatrics* 1998;102:346-354.

4.   Berman S: Otitis media in children. *N Engl J Med* 1995; 332:1560-1565.

5.   American Academy of Pediatrics, The Otitis Media Guideline Panel: Managing otitis media with effusion in young children. *Pediatrics* 1994;94:766-773.

6.   Lildholdt T, Cantekin EI, Bluestone CD, et al: Effect of topical nasal decongestant on eustachian tube function in children with tympanostomy tubes. *Acta Otolaryngol (Stockh)* 1982;94:93-97.

7.   Bess FH, Tharpe AM: Unilateral hearing impairment in children. *Pediatrics* 1984;74:206-216.

8.   Holm VA, Kunze LH: Effect of chronic otitis media on language and speech development. *Pediatrics* 1969;43:833-839.

9.   Kaplan GJ, Fleshman JK, Bender TR, et al: Long-term effects of otitis media: a ten-year cohort study of Alaskan Eskimo children. *Pediatrics* 1973;52:577-585.

10. Lewis N: Otitis media and linguistic incompetence. *Arch Otolaryngol* 1976;102:387-390.

11. Needleman H: Effects of hearing loss from recurrent otitis media on speech and language development. In: Jaffe BF, ed. *Hearing Loss in Children*. Baltimore, University Park Press, 1977, pp 640-649.

12. Sak RJ, Ruben RJ: Recurrent middle ear effusion in childhood: implications of temporary auditory deprivation for language and learning. *Ann Otol Rhinol Laryngol* 1981;90:546-551.

13. Friel-Patti S, Finitzo-Hieber T, Conti G, et al: Language delay in infants associated with middle ear disease and mild, fluctuating hearing impairment. *Pediatr Infect Dis* 1982;1:104-109.

14. Teele DW, Klein JO, Rosner BA: Otitis media with effusion during the first three years of life and development of speech and language. *Pediatrics* 1984;74:282-287.

15. Teele DW, Klein JO, Chase C, et al: Otitis media in infancy and intellectual ability, school achievement, speech, and language at age 7 years. Greater Boston Otitis Media Study Group. *J Infect Dis* 1990;162:685-694.

16. Wright PF, Sell SH, McConnell KB, et al: Impact of recurrent otitis media on middle ear function, hearing, and language. *J Pediatr* 1988;113:581-587.

17. Roberts JE, Burchinal MR, Medley LP, et al: Otitis media, hearing sensitivity, and maternal responsiveness in relation to language during infancy. *J Pediatr* 1995;126:481-489.

18. Feagans L, Fipp E, Blood I: The effect of otitis media on the attention skills of day-care-attending toddlers. *Dev Psychol* 1994;30:701-708.

19. Wallace IF, Gravel JS, Schwartz RG, et al: Otitis media, communication style of primary caregivers, and language skills of 2-year-olds: a preliminary report. *J Dev Behav Pediatr* 1996;17: 27-35.

20. Black MM, Sonnenschein S: Early exposure to otitis media: a preliminary investigation of behavioral outcome. *J Dev Behav Pediatr* 1993;14:150-155.

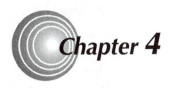

Chapter 4

Microbiology

The organisms causing acute otitis media (AOM) have remained relatively constant the past 2 decades. *Streptococcus pneumoniae* is responsible for 25% to 50% of cases; nontypeable *Haemophilus influenzae*, 15% to 30%; *Moraxella catarrhalis*, 3% to 20%; and viral etiologies account for 15% to 25%[1,2] (Figure 1 and Table 1). However, the susceptibility of these pathogenic bacteria to usual outpatient antimicrobial therapy has significantly changed; resistance to amoxicillin, the previously recommended first-line therapy, is increasingly prevalent. Clinicians were warned a decade ago that β-lactamase production by *H influenzae* and *M catarrhalis* was common. By the late 1990s, 40% to 50% of *H influenzae* and 90% to 100% of *M catarrhalis* were not susceptible to amoxicillin because of this mechanism. More importantly, *S pneumoniae* has now developed amoxicillin resistance via an alteration in penicillin-binding proteins (PBP), which also renders these organisms nonsusceptible to penicillin/β-lactamase inhibitor combinations such as amoxicillin/clavulanate (Augmentin®) and ticarcillin/clavulanate (Timentin®).[3]

These changes in susceptibility patterns for organisms causing AOM once again raise the question considered periodically over the past 20 years: is amoxicillin still the drug of choice for AOM? Today, more data compel consideration of other classes of antibiotics for primary therapy. Macrolides (eg, azithromycin [Zithromax®], clarithromycin [Biaxin®], erythromycin), most cepha-

49

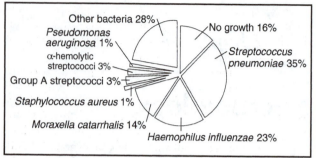

Figure 1: Pathogens recovered by tympanocentesis from the middle ear fluid of 2,807 patients with AOM. These studies were done at the Pittsburgh Otitis Media Center, and include patients who underwent tympanocentesis between 1980 and 1989 (total percentages exceed 100% because multiple bacteria were recovered from some patients).[1,2]

Table 1: Bacterial Pathogens Isolated From Middle Ear Fluids in Children With AOM[2]

Pathogen	Mean (%)	Range (%)
S pneumoniae	39	27-52
H influenzae	27	16-52
M catarrhalis	10	2-27
Streptococcus pyogenes	3	0-11
None or nonpathogens	30	12-45

losporins, particularly cefprozil (Cefzil®), cefpodoxime proxetil (Vantin®), and loracarbef (Lorabid®, actually a carbacephem antibiotic) all have excellent activity against penicillin-resistant pneumococci and β-lactamase-producing *H influenzae* and *M catarrhalis*. The increased dosage recommendations for amoxicillin and amoxicillin/clavulanate (Chapter 6) also cover a higher percentage of amoxicillin-resistant *S pneumoniae*.

Physicians must select first-line therapy for otitis media based on regional susceptibility data of bacterial pathogens and, more importantly, on documented treatment failure rates of previous regimens. Regional differences for these variables make it difficult to offer recommendations that are appropriate for all locations. If a decision is made to change from amoxicillin (or trimethoprim/sulfamethoxazole [Bactrim™, Septra®, TMP/SMX]) as first-line therapy, there are many options (see Chapter 6). Other considerations for selection might include cost and compliance issues. Compliance is enhanced for antibiotics that taste better, that are given once or twice rather than 3 or 4 times a day, and that are given for lesser durations.

A change from amoxicillin to other classes of antibiotics for most outpatient infections also offers the theoretic advantage of reversing the trend to penicillin resistance among common pathogens by eliminating the pressure for mutation that always occurs with excessive use of a single agent.[4] A change in present strategy may yield the opportunity to return to amoxicillin in the future.

Etiology of AOM
Streptococcus pneumoniae
Pneumococci remain the most common bacterial pathogens causing AOM. A recent and relatively rapid change in antimicrobial sensitivity pattern causes great concern—specifically, high-level resistance to penicillin along with resistance to other classes of antibiotics, including cephalosporins, macrolides, TMP/SMX, and chloramphenicol.[3,4]

Unlike most other forms of resistance to penicillin or other β-lactam antibiotics, which are mediated by β-lactamase production, pneumococci have developed mechanisms for altering PBPs to avert killing by antimicrobial agents. PBPs comprise six high-molecular-weight enzymes, designated 1A, 1B, 2A, 2B, 2X, and 3, that are located in the cell wall of many bacterial species.

Cell wall enzymes synthesize peptidoglycan, which is essential for the building and modification of bacterial cell walls. These enzymes also provide the binding sites for penicillin and other β-lactam antibiotics. The main attachment site for penicillin is PBP2B. If penicillin cannot bind to the organism, subsequent steps in antimicrobial activity are prevented.

Laboratory studies have shown that sustained exposure of penicillin-susceptible pneumococci to gradually increasing concentrations of penicillin results in the selection of stable resistant mutants because of the reduced binding capacity of PBPs. This process increases the concentrations of antibiotic needed for bacterial killing.

Chromosomal gene alterations are primarily responsible for the changes in PBPs. Because PBP is an enzyme that has undergone change, resistance is further enhanced because of altered peptidoglycan-branched peptide patterns within a newly modified cell wall, which are not easily disrupted by the usual mechanisms of penicillin.

Laboratory strains of pneumococci during the 1940s showed that resistance can be transferred by the DNA material of many streptococcal organisms (interspecies), as well as by other related pneumococci (intraspecies). These genetic mutations usually occur independently, resulting in heterogeneous resistance patterns.

Analysis of PBPs of these resistant organisms demonstrates that they do not represent the same mutations, since alterations in PBPs are highly variable. However, well-documented examples show spread of a single clone mutant from one country to another. An outbreak of penicillin-resistant pneumococcal disease in Spain was shown to be caused by organisms possessing a single PBP change identical to strains causing an outbreak in South Africa. During a similar cluster of cases in the United States, most isolates had an identical alteration, suggesting that these strains were related to those in the earlier outbreaks in Europe and South Africa.

Recent surveys have also demonstrated that pneumococcal colonization in young infants is related to duration of attendance in child-care centers. A survey of these facilities in Louisiana found that pneumococcal colonization rates were 50% for children who attended less than 20 hours a week, but were almost 85% among those who attended more than 20 hours.[2] The predominant pneumococcal serotypes colonizing these children were 3, 6, 9, 14, 19, and 23, which are also the serotypes that cause OM.

Another important recent observation is that most pneumococcal OM occurs within 1 month after a child becomes colonized with a new strain of *S pneumoniae*. The attack rate has been shown to be about 15% during this critical period.[5] The colonizing pneumococci remain for 1 to 2 months, after which another may take its place. The child's environment likely determines the organisms that inhabit the posterior nasopharynx and, in homes or day-care centers with a high prevalence of amoxicillin-resistant pneumococci, colonization is more likely to occur with organisms that require other antibiotics for treatment. This epidemiologic information is obviously important in managing new episodes of AOM.

Nosocomial infections have been described, including AOM with both penicillin-resistant and multidrug-resistant pneumococci. Predisposing factors include prolonged duration of hospitalization and nasopharyngeal carriage. One study reported that 35% of children hospitalized longer than 14 days became colonized with multiresistant strains prevalent in the hospital, and overt infection developed in some of these patients.[6] The most common areas for hospital transmission of disease are intensive care units.

Identifying Pneumococcal Resistance. The National Committee for Clinical Laboratory Standards (NCCLS) defines susceptibility of *S pneumoniae* to penicillin as a minimum inhibitory concentration (MIC) of equal to or less than 0.06 µg/mL. The definition of intermediate resistance is an MIC of 0.1 to 1 µg/mL; an MIC of 2 µg/mL or more defines highly resistant strains. The 2 µg/mL breakpoint for penicillin is appropriate for AOM because it is difficult to achieve higher levels of the drug in middle ear fluid.

Screening for penicillin resistance can be easily achieved with a 1-µg oxacillin disk placed on a Mueller-Hinton sheep agar plate containing test organisms. A disk zone diameter of 19 mm or less defines potential resistance. A methicillin disk may also be used; with this disk a zone diameter of 25 mm or less defines resistance.

The oxacillin disk produces results within 24 hours. The specificity of this method is 90% to 95%, and the sensitivity is over 99%, so this is quite adequate as a screening standard. As with any screening test, all potentially resistant isolates must be tested using a quantitative MIC assay to confirm susceptibility. A small but significant percentage of organisms with an inhibition zone around the oxacillin disk of 19 mm or less are still susceptible to penicillin. Almost all of these have zone sizes of 17 to 19 mm.

There are numerous methods for definitive sensitivity testing, including Kirby-Bauer disk dilution, broth macrodilution, broth microdilution, agar dilution, and the newly developed epsilometric (E) test. For broth dilution testing, the recommended medium is Mueller-Hinton broth with 5% lysed centrifuged horse blood; however, this is not commercially available and is relatively difficult to prepare. Appropriate training is therefore essential.

Repetitive testing for susceptibility is best achieved with either the broth microdilution assay or the E test; both provide specific inhibitory concentrations. The E test is a relatively expensive but very simple method that requires little technician time. This test uses a paper strip that has been impregnated with a linear concentration gradient of

Table 2: NCCLS Guidelines for Susceptibility of *S pneumoniae*, March 1999

Antibiotic	MIC ($\leq\mu$g/mL)
amoxicillin	2
amoxicillin/clavulanate	2
azithromycin	0.5
cefaclor	8
cefixime	1
cefotaxime*	1
cefpodoxime proxetil	0.5
ceftriaxone*	0.5
cefuroxime axetil	1
chloramphenicol	4
clarithromycin	0.25
clindamycin	0.25
erythromycin	0.5
loracarbef	8
penicillin*	0.06
trimethoprim/sulfamethoxazole	0.5
vancomycin	1

*2 μg/mL or more for cefotaxime, ceftriaxone, or penicillin indicates high resistance

the antibiotic being assayed. The paper strip is placed directly on the agar plate containing the organisms, and the antibiotic is released into the agar matrix at the same gradient of concentrations contained on the strip.

Multiple E-test strips for different antibiotics can be placed on the same agar plate. The MIC is read directly on the strip where it crosses the narrowing zone of bacterial growth.

Multidrug resistance is defined as resistance to three or more antibiotics of different classes (those with different mechanisms of action). For cefotaxime (Claforan®) and ceftriaxone (Rocephin®), the NCCLS has proposed breakpoints of 1 µg/mL and 0.5 µg/mL, respectively, for intermediate resistance, and 2 µg/mL or more for high resistance. Susceptibility and resistance breakpoints for other antibiotics are presented in Table 2.

Pneumococcal strains that are highly resistant to penicillin are much more likely to be resistant to other antibiotics, particularly cephalosporins. Surveillance data for pneumococci colonizing the posterior nasopharynx of young children indicate that approximately 10% of strains with an MIC of 2 µg/mL or more for penicillin are also resistant to cefotaxime. All strains that are susceptible or intermediately resistant to penicillin are generally sensitive to most cephalosporins and many other classes of antibiotics. The degree of penicillin resistance is therefore an important marker for predicting broad-spectrum resistance patterns.

The emergence of multiple-resistant organisms has obvious clinical implications. Antibiotic resistance and the increased prevalence of β-lactamase-producing *H influenzae* and *Moraxella catarrhalis* now challenge the traditional recommendation for using amoxicillin as the antibiotic of choice for many outpatient infections, particularly ear infections.

Haemophilus influenzae

Clinicians must recognize that 90% to 95% of *H influenzae* in AOM are nontypeable strains. This is why the introduction of *H influenzae* type B vaccine has had no impact on the frequency of *H influenzae* OM. The incidence of OM caused by this organism actually increased during the 1990s after the *H influenzae* vaccine was introduced. The reason for the increase is not related to the vaccine but rather to other factors, particularly day-care center attendance during this decade.

Nontypeable *H influenzae* commonly colonizes the posterior nasopharynx in young children, which largely accounts for its ranking as the second most common organism associated with both OM and sinusitis. Nontypeable *H influenzae* also account for the conjunctivitis-OM syndrome. The recognition of this combination infection is important for anticipating specific organisms that are involved in middle ear disease. *H influenzae* can be recovered from cultures of conjunctival exudate and susceptibilities determined for guiding therapy if routine antibiotics are ineffective.

At present, 40% to 50% of nontypeable strains of *H influenzae* produce β-lactamase, which makes them resistant to amoxicillin and other penicillins that do not contain β-lactamase inhibitors.

Moraxella catarrhalis

Before the early 1980s, *M catarrhalis* was rarely reported as a cause of AOM. However, during the past 2 decades this pathogen has emerged as the third most common cause of ear infections, replacing group A β-hemolytic streptococci, which now account for only 3% of cases. *M catarrhalis* organisms have two unique characteristics important in the clinical management of AOM: (1) an almost absolute prevalence of β-lactamase production; and (2) a high propensity for spontaneous resolution. These factors greatly affect the selection of first-line therapy for AOM and considerations for delayed antimicrobial therapy.

M catarrhalis demonstrates few virulence characteristics, resulting in its rare identification in cases of invasive bacterial disease. For this reason, it was initially surprising that it was a common cause of AOM. Early reservations about its pathogenicity were eliminated when serologic studies clearly showed a rise in immunoglobulin G (IgG) and immunoglobulin A (IgA) antibodies in both serum and middle ear fluids during the course of middle ear disease, only when *M catarrhalis* was recovered from middle ear exudate. These data have documented causality and pathogenicity.

During the 1960s, all strains of *M catarrhalis* were susceptible to amoxicillin (penicillin). By 1990, more than 75% of these strains produced β-lactamase, and were therefore resistant to all penicillins. This observation, along with the increased β-lactamase production by *H influenzae*, led to the increased use of amoxicillin/clavulanate as first-line therapy for AOM. At present, virtually all *M catarrhalis* produce β-lactamase, while one half of all *H influenzae* generate this enzyme. Along with the increased amoxicillin resistance among pneumococci, which results from a change in penicillin-binding proteins rather than β-lactamase production, amoxicillin appears to be a poor choice as first-line therapy for all AOM.

The other interesting characteristic of *M catarrhalis* is its high incidence of spontaneous resolution, observed in more than 70% of patients who received placebo or ineffective antibiotics during controlled clinical trials. This high rate of spontaneous cure, which likely results from relatively low virulence among these organisms, has increased support for the option of delayed therapy in AOM (Chapter 7). Obviously, if this pathogen could be predicted, fewer than 1 in 3 children would require antimicrobial therapy. Unfortunately, without tympanocentesis, etiology cannot be predicted.

Other Bacteria

Other pathogens consistently recovered from 1% to 3% of patients in AOM studies where tympanocentesis was performed are group A streptococci, *Staphylococcus aureus*, and anaerobic bacteria. Before 1970, group A *Streptococcus* was the second or third most common cause of AOM according to various published series, accounting for 10% to 15% of infection, but for unexplained reasons is now recovered much less frequently.

The importance of anaerobes in AOM and OME has long been debated, but most experts feel that their role is limited. *Peptostreptococcus* has been most frequently isolated in AOM, and has been identified along with *Fusobacterium* and *Bacteroides* in studies of OME.

Chlamydia pneumoniae has recently emerged as an organism that may cause a significant percentage of middle ear infections, perhaps accounting for many of the cases previously considered culture negative. Newer culture and antigen detection techniques are being used to better define the relevance of this potential pathogen.

Viral Etiologies

Viruses play a significant role in the pathogenesis of AOM, both as primary etiologic pathogens and as initiators of inflammatory responses that augment bacterial replication[7] (Table 3). The incidence of AOM clearly increases during outbreaks of viral infection, particularly those caused by respiratory syncytial virus (RSV), but also is well documented with rhinovirus, influenza, parainfluenza, and adenovirus disease.[8] Inflammation produced by these viral infections progresses to eustachian tube obstruction, serous fluid accumulation, and subsequent growth of colonizing bacteria within the middle ear cavity. During the progression of these events, responsible viruses can be cultured from the throat, posterior nasopharynx, and from the middle ear itself. This pattern has been documented in more than 25% of AOM cases in children younger than 3 years. The most convincing studies isolated viruses or viral antigens from middle ear fluids. With newer virus identification techniques, more than 1 in 6 cases of AOM have been shown to be associated with

Table 3: Viral Isolates From Children With AOM[7]

Virus	Middle Ear Fluid (%)	Nasopharynx (%)
Respiratory syncytial virus	7	15
Rhinovirus	3	14
Influenza virus	2	2
Adenovirus	2	5
Parainfluenza viruses	1	2
Enteroviruses	1	1
Rotavirus	0	0
Total	17	39

middle ear viral colonization, most in conjunction with bacterial pathogens. Twice this number of documented bacterial ear infections occur in association with nasopharyngeal viral disease. During outbreaks of RSV infection, this association is much greater: in 64% of all bacterial AOM cases, RSV can be isolated from the upper respiratory tract or middle ear.[9] RSV as a predisposing factor to AOM is even more apparent in studies that have examined the natural history of RSV disease in infants. Two thirds of all RSV-infected children develop AOM during the course of infection, a sufficiently high incidence to support routine antimicrobial therapy once RSV is identified in children with symptomatic pulmonary disease.

When viral and bacterial pathogens coexist, treatment with antibiotics results in slower resolution and a higher frequency of both microbiologic and clinical failures, compared with disease produced by bacteria alone. Recent data suggest that this may result from decreased penetration of antibiotics into the middle ear, attributable to the presence of viral pathogens and viral-induced inflammatory changes.[10]

Because RSV is essentially a universal infection during childhood, it is the most common virus recovered from the middle ear and nasopharynx in most studies of AOM that have included culture data. Although RSV is the only pathogen isolated in 5% to 6% of patients with AOM, it is identified along with one of the common bacterial organisms twice as often. This suggests that an effective vaccine for RSV may lower the incidence of AOM. Passive immunization with intravenous RSV immunoglobulin has been shown to provide this preventive effect.

Rhinovirus, second only to RSV as a potential AOM pathogen, will be more difficult to control with vaccines because many strains have been identified and immunity after infection appears to be brief. Some experts recommend administering prophylactic antibiotics for the duration of rhinovirus-induced upper respiratory infections to prevent secondary bacterial AOM.

During outbreaks of viral disease, particularly during the annual winter epidemics of RSV, this organism is often the most common documented cause of middle ear disease. Likewise, influenza and parainfluenza viruses are significant when respiratory infection caused by these agents is prevalent. The association between influenza viruses and secondary bacterial AOM is so common that some experts have suggested routine influenza immunizations to reduce the incidence of AOM, particularly for children who are prone to OM.

Organisms Associated with OME

Although, by definition, children with otitis media with effusion (OME) do not have fever or other symptoms suggesting overt infection, bacteria have been recovered from about half of these patients when tympanocentesis was performed.[2] This has been a consistent observation, even when effusions have been present for more than 2 months.

Unfortunately, neither differences in the characteristics of middle ear fluid nor other variables on examination of the tympanic membrane identify those patients with bacterial infection. Decisions for management of OME, including repeat courses of antibiotics, must therefore apply to all patients, including those who may have sterile effusions.

Pathogens tend to be similar to those causing AOM, with *H influenzae*, *S pneumoniae*, and *M catarrhalis* accounting for approximately 50% of all isolates. As contrasted with AOM, *H influenzae* appears to be somewhat more prevalent than pneumococci. The greatest difference from AOM in all published series is the much higher recovery of organisms generally considered nonvirulent. These include *Staphylococcus epidermidis*, nonhemolytic and microaerophilic streptococci, *Propionibacterium acnes*, and diphtheroids. Such bacteria are unlikely to cause recurrence of acute middle ear infection. Therefore, only 10% to 25% of OME cases potentially need additional antimicrobial therapy.

Neonatal Pathogens

The etiology of neonatal OM is unique because a significant percentage of disease is caused by gram-negative coliform bacilli, and a small percentage by group B streptococci and *S aureus*[11-14] (Table 4). Still, more than half of pathogens are those normally seen in older children: *S pneumoniae* and *H influenzae* are the first and second most commonly isolated bacteria. Because of the unique antimicrobial susceptibility patterns for enteric bacteria, it becomes more important to establish the etiology of cases in neonates. Some experts recommend routine tympanocentesis in this age group. Others point out that because most of these cases can be treated with the usual antibiotics, tympanocentesis can be reserved for children who fail therapy after 48 to 72 hours of treatment and careful monitoring. These children are then most appropriately man-

Table 4: Bacterial Pathogens Causing AOM During the First 6 Weeks of Life[11-14]

Microorganism	Percentage of Infants with Pathogen
S pneumoniae	18
H influenzae	12
S aureus	8
Escherichia coli	6
M catarrhalis	5
Klebsiella and Enterobacter species	5
S pneumoniae and H influenzae	3
Streptococcus, groups A and B	3
Pseudomonas aeruginosa	2
Miscellaneous	5
None or nonpathogens	32

aged with the help of an otolaryngologic surgeon so that a carefully performed tympanocentesis can be done. If gram-negative organisms or gram-positive cocci in clusters are observed in tympanocentesis fluid, indicating a coliform or staphylococcal etiology, antibiotics can be appropriately adjusted. These infants should be managed in the hospital with parenteral therapy guided by susceptibility data from isolated organisms. Many experts recommend examination of the cerebrospinal fluid (CSF) before beginning parenteral antibiotics, particularly if the patient manifests any evidence of toxicity. These young patients have a higher predisposition to chronic middle ear disease and extension into the mastoid air cells or central nervous system. Long-term follow-up is therefore warranted.

Organisms Causing
Chronic Suppurative Otitis Media

Chronic suppurative otitis media (CSOM) is a sequela of poorly responsive recurrent AOM with a perforation of the tympanic membrane that persists for more than 6 weeks. Exudative and serous fluid in the middle ear and external canal supports replication of colonizing microbial flora, particularly *Pseudomonas aeruginosa* and *S aureus*.[15] These are the same organisms that cause external otitis, whose pathogenesis is similar to CSOM except that the tympanic membrane is not perforated. Additional organisms occasionally recovered from exudative material are gram-negative coliforms, anaerobes, and atypical mycobacteria. Most other common bacterial flora of the external ear canal do not appear to be pathogenic, and thus can generally be disregarded when recovered in cultures of ear drainage. These include *S epidermidis*, diphtheroids, *P acnes*, and anaerobic cocci.

Multiple virulence factors associated with *Pseudomonas* and *S aureus* account for persistent and sometimes progressive middle ear disease. Aggressive medical management is therefore warranted, often requiring parenteral therapy. Cultures of exudative material, with identification of pathogens and their susceptibilities, best direct appropriate antimicrobial therapy. The *Pseudomonas* and *S aureus* strains recovered from these patients tend to be sensitive organisms, although in the case of *Pseudomonas*, only fluoroquinolones are effective as oral therapy, and these are not approved for use in children. However, newer topical quinolones are safe and effective for the treatment of CSOM in children (see Chapter 6).

Organisms Causing Mastoiditis

Mastoiditis is an infection of the posterior process of the temporal bone, almost exclusively a consequence of prolonged middle ear suppuration. Disease may evolve with either acute or chronic manifestations, and these two presentations are distinctly different in bacterial etiology. Thus, pathogens recovered in cases of acute mastoiditis reflect those that more commonly cause AOM, while the etiologic agents of chronic mastoiditis are identical to those in CSOM. Combining data for acute mastoiditis from studies published between 1980 and 1996, the most commonly recovered microorganisms were *S pneumoniae* (29%), *Streptococcus pyogenes* (22%), and *S aureus* (17%).[16] Bacteria causing chronic mastoiditis in the same period were predominantly *P aeruginosa*, *S aureus*, and a variety of anaerobic organisms.

Recent reports have identified nontuberculous mycobacteria as a cause of chronic mastoiditis in children.[16] A cluster of 17 cases of OM, including three with mastoiditis caused by *Mycobacterium chelonei* resulting from contamination of otologic instruments in a single office, was the largest series of nontuberculous ear disease in the United States. Other reports have been from scattered cases, attesting to the rarity of middle ear infections caused by these pathogens. Three recent cases of mastoiditis in immunocompetent Swedish children included the first caused by *M kansasii* and another caused by *M abscessus*, previously named *M chelonei* subspecies *abscessus*. These cases were important in defining the need for combined surgical and medical management. Revision mastoidectomies were necessary in all patients, and antimicrobial therapy for *M abscessus* and *M chelonei* required extensive susceptibility testing to all classes of potentially useful agents.

References

1. Steele RW: Management of otitis media. *Infect Med* 1998; 15:174-178, 203.

2. Bluestone CD, Stephenson JS, Martin LM: Ten-year review of otitis media pathogens. *Pediatr Infect Dis J* 1992;11:S7-S11.

3. Steele RW, Warrier R, Unkel PJ, et al: Colonization with antibiotic-resistant *Streptococcus pneumoniae* in children with sickle cell disease. *J Pediatr* 1996;128:531-535.

4. Steele RW: Drug-resistant pneumococci. *J Resp Dis* 1995;16: 624-633.

5. Gray BM, Converse GM 3rd, Dillon HC Jr: Epidemiologic studies of *Streptococcus pneumoniae* in infants: acquisition, carriage, and infection during the first 24 months of life. *J Infect Dis* 1980;142:923-933.

6. Breiman RF, Butler JC, Tenover FL, et al: Emergence of drug-resistant pneumococcal infections in the United States. *JAMA* 1994;271:1831-1835.

7. Ruuskanen O, Arola M, Heikkinen T, et al: Viruses in acute otitis media: increasing evidence for clinical significance. *Pediatr Infect Dis J* 1991;10:425-427.

8. Pitkaranta A, Virolainen A, Jero J, et al: Detection of rhinovirus, respiratory syncytial virus, and coronavirus infections in acute otitis media by reverse transcriptase polymerase chain reaction. *Pediatrics* 1998;102:291-295.

9. Okamoto Y, Kudo K, Ishikawa K, et al: Presence of respiratory syncytial virus genomic sequences in middle ear fluid and its relationship to expression of cytokines and cell adhesion molecules. *J Infect Dis* 1993;168:1277-1281.

10. Canafax DM, Yuan Z, Chonmaitree T, et al: Amoxicillin middle ear fluid penetration and pharmacokinetics in children with acute otitis media. *Pediatr Infect Dis J* 1998;17:149-156.

11. Berman SA, Balkany TJ, Simmons MA: Otitis media in the neonatal intensive care unit. *Pediatrics* 1978;62:198-201.

12. Bland RD: Otitis media in the first six weeks of life: diagnosis, bacteriology, and management. *Pediatrics* 1972;49:187-197.

13. Shurin PA, Howie VM, Pelton SI, et al: Bacterial etiology of otitis media during the first six weeks of life. *J Pediatr* 1978;92: 893-896.

14. Tetzlaff TR, Ashworth C, Nelson JD: Otitis media in children less than 12 weeks of age. *Pediatrics* 1977;59:827-832.

15. Kenna MA, Bluestone CD, Reilly JS, et al: Medical management of chronic suppurative otitis media without cholesteatoma in children. *Laryngoscope* 1986;96:146-151.

16. Bitar CN, Kluka EA, Steele RW: Mastoiditis in children. *Clin Pediatr (Phila)* 1996;35:391-395.

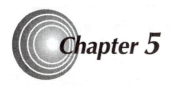

Chapter 5

Otoscopy, Acoustic Immittance, and Audiometry

Proper evaluation of a child with recurrent otitis media (OM) depends on the medical history, physical examination, and, at times, acoustic immittance and audiology. The physical examination focuses on the otologic evaluation, specifically pneumatic otoscopy. A complete examination of the child should be performed because it may provide insight into predisposing factors for recurrent infections. Examination of the child should therefore include notation of craniofacial anomalies, cleft palate or submucous cleft, allergic facies, and adenoid hypertrophy.

Physical Examination and Otoscopy

In addition to an inspection of the tympanic membrane (TM), the otologic examination should include evaluation of the auricle and external auditory canal. Evidence of postauricular erythema and edema, discharge within the external auditory canal, and TM integrity should all be noted. Pneumatic otoscopy is integral to any otologic examination and provides invaluable, essential information about the status of both the TM and middle ear; the examination is incomplete without it.

Unfortunately, obtaining an adequate otologic view, especially in the pediatric population, may be very diffi-

Table 1: Difficult Otologic Examinations

- Moving target (inadequate immobilization)
- Blocked view (cerumen in the external auditory canal)
- Inadequate equipment (poor illumination)

cult. Challenges in this population include the patient (the 'moving target' phenomenon), the ear canal (a cerumen impaction), or inadequate equipment (Table 1). Although the examination of a cooperative child may be relatively effortless, children who have had previous sensitization (ie, previous otologic trauma) rarely acquiesce easily, despite significant coaxing and bribing. Adequate otologic visualization in these 'sensitized' infants and children often requires significant immobilization. If a 'good look' is all that is necessary, the child may be stabilized in the mother's 'grip' with one hand holding the child's head, one arm stabilizing the child's arms, and the mother's thighs gripping the child's legs (Figure 1).

If cerumen or a foreign body exists within the meatus, a more controlled restraint technique, involving either a papoose or human restraint on an examining chair or table, may be required (Figure 2). When physical restraint is impossible, such as with larger or neurologically impaired children, a trial of Debrox® with reassessment or examination under general anesthesia may be required. Cerumen removal may be accomplished with a cerumen loop or small suction, using an otoscope with a surgical head or a microscope. Some clinicians advocate 'flushing' with a dental irrigator. This should be performed cautiously, especially if there is any potential for a TM perforation or if a tympanostomy tube is in place. During cerumen removal, the child must be com-

Figure 1A/B:
The mother's 'grip'.

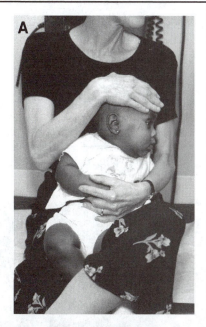

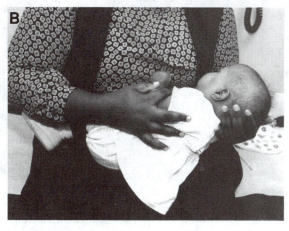

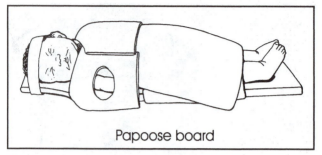

Papoose board

Figure 2: *Papoosing.*

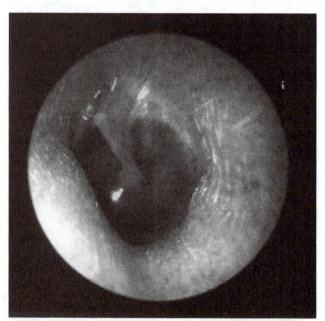

Figure 3: *Normal tympanic membrane. Used with permission from Handler S, Myers C:* Ear, Nose, and Throat Disease in Children. *Hamilton, Ontario, BC Decker, 1998.*

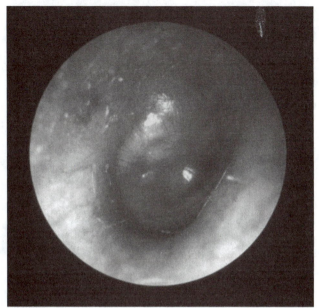

Figure 4: *Acute otitis media. Used with permission from Handler S, Myers C:* Ear, Nose, and Throat Disease in Children. *Hamilton, Ontario, BC Decker, 1998.*

pletely immobilized. Contact with the exquisitely sensitive external canal often results in abrupt movements and consequent otologic trauma.

Pneumatic otoscopy provides visualization and dynamic understanding of the TM and middle ear status. Proper equipment is essential. The diagnostic head must provide adequate illumination and magnification. The largest speculum that comfortably fits in the canal should provide an airtight seal. The TM is initially assessed for its position, color, translucency, and mobility. A normal TM is translucent, concave, and pearly gray (Figure 3). A healthy TM offers a view of many middle ear structures, including the malleus, incudostapedial joint, promontory,

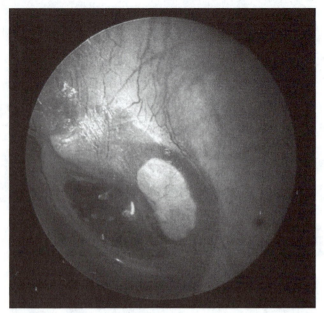

Figure 5: *Tympanosclerosis. Used with permission from Handler S, Myers C:* Ear, Nose, and Throat Disease in Children. *Hamilton, Ontario, BC Decker, 1998.*

and occasionally the round window niche (Figure 3). In a healthy ear, the TM is briskly mobile; the mobility of the TM reflects the status of both the middle ear and the TM. Decreased mobility indicates increased impedance or fluid within the middle ear, a stiff TM, or an inadequate seal. Pneumatic otoscopy is less accurate in infants because their pliable external canals distend and collapse with insufflation, while their TMs are positioned in a more horizontal plane, making them appear smaller and retracted.

In the early stages of acute otitis media (AOM), the TM becomes hyperemic, and a purulent effusion develops. The TM bulges, becoming opaque with decreased mobility (Figure 4). In a crying child, the TM may also

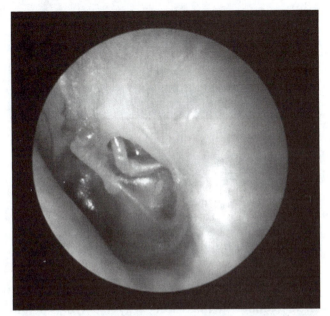

Figure 6: Myringostapediopexy. Used with permission from Handler S, Myers C: Ear, Nose, and Throat Disease in Children. Hamilton, Ontario, BC Decker, 1998.

become hyperemic secondary to vascular engorgement, although normal mobility is evident on pneumatic otoscopy. With the resolution of AOM, a serous effusion often remains. This is seen as a retracted, dull TM with decreased mobility, or a full TM with an air-fluid level. Development of negative middle ear pressure results in a retracted TM with a foreshortened malleus.

A TM that has sustained recurrent or continuous middle ear inflammation becomes thickened or infiltrated with a tympanosclerotic plaque, ie, calcium deposits within the middle layer of the TM (Figure 5). These pathologic changes within the TM obscure the normal middle ear landmarks, decrease its mobility, and imply

- Tympanogram
- Stapedial reflexes
- Equivalent ear-canal volume

a history of chronic infections. Atelectasis or retraction of the TM may occur in an environment of prolonged negative middle ear pressure. *Atelectasis* refers to an atrophic drum with an incompletely expanded middle ear space; *retraction* refers to medial displacement of the TM. Diffuse retraction and atrophy often are used interchangeably. The mobility of the atelectatic TM varies from a hyperdynamic piece of 'cellophane' to the immobility of 'shrink wrap.' As the atelectasis becomes more adhesive, the TM adheres to the middle ear structures, creating a myringoincudopexy (incus) or a myringostapediopexy (incudostapedial joint) (Figure 6). A localized retraction of the TM may result in bottlenecking (a retraction pocket), evolving into a sac and ultimately into a destructive cholesteatoma.

Acoustic Immittance

While pneumatic otoscopy is subjective and often imprecise, acoustic immittance offers an objective method of evaluating middle ear status. Acoustic immittance requires no active participation by the patient, and may provide three points of data: the tympanogram, the stapedial reflexes, and the equivalent ear-canal volume (Table 2). The tympanogram is the most common test, providing a graphic display of TM impedance. The Y axis records TM compliance, and the X axis records pressure in millimeters of water. A probe inserted into the external meatus changes the ear canal pressure from positive to negative,

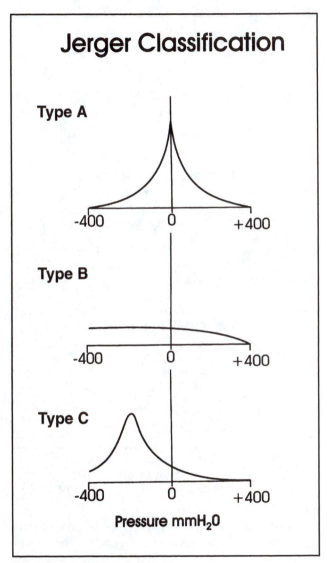

Figure 7: Jerger classification.

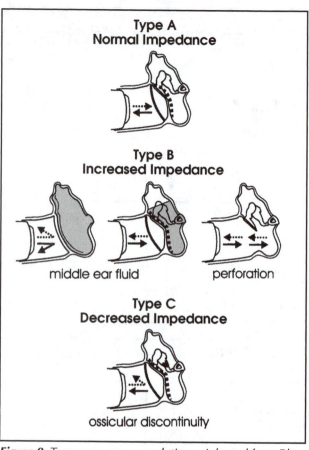

Figure 8: *Tympanogram correlations. Adapted from Blue-stone CD, Klein JO, eds:* Otitis Media in Infants and Children, *2nd ed. Philadelphia, WB Saunders, 1995.*

varying the stiffness of the TM. The reflected energy or signal from the TM is measured and recorded. The signal's amplitude and phase are determined by the mechanical properties of the TM.

In a normal tympanogram, where middle ear pressure is equivalent to atmospheric pressure, a peak is demonstrated at approximately 0 mm H_2O. In negative middle ear pressure, a peak is demonstrated in the negative pressure zone. The height of the peak also indicates the impedance of the TM-middle ear system. A hypermobile TM with decreased impedance demonstrates an elevated peak. In contrast, an increase in impedance, as in middle ear effusion, is demonstrated by a decreased peak or a flat line.

The accuracy, ease, and affordability of tympanometry have led to its widespread use in clinical screening. Jerger has classified three basic tympanometric patterns: A, B, and C (Figure 7). Type A tympanogram, indicative of normal middle ear pressure, has a peak between -100 and 0 mm H_2O (Figure 8). Type B tympanogram has either a flat or a very round peak, and is usually consistent with middle ear effusion or TM perforation. Type C tympanogram has a sharp peak below -150 mm H_2O, and indicates negative middle ear pressure. A type C tympanogram, especially with pressures less than -250 mm H_2O, may have a coexistent middle ear effusion. Studies have demonstrated a high level of accuracy between tympanometry and myringotomy findings, although certain clinical findings have demonstrated some variability, especially in conjunction with negative middle ear pressure.

In infants younger than 7 months, tympanometry is not accurate because of the hypercompliant nature of the external ear canal. Traditional tympanometry uses a single tone frequency at 220 or 226 Hz and measures a 'single-peaked' graph. Tympanometry in infants produces a double-peaked graph, making its interpretation extremely difficult. Tympanograms that measure a spectrum of frequencies, rather than a single frequency, provide more information about middle ear resonance, especially in infants younger than 4 months. The use of high-frequency tones, 660 or 800 Hz, is especially sensitive to middle ear status in infants, and can distinguish between normal infant ears and those with effusions.

Acoustic immittance may also estimate equivalent ear canal volume, ie, volume of air lateral to the TM. The normal volume of air lateral to an intact TM is 0.5 to 1 mL in a young child; the volume in an adult or older child is 0.65 to 1.75 mL. Equivalent ear canal volume is larger in a perforated TM than in an intact TM. This becomes significant in evaluation of a type B (flat) tympanogram and in the differentiation between a middle ear effusion and a perforated TM (myringotomy tube). Equivalent ear canal volumes are not accurate in a canal wall down mastoidectomies.

Demonstration of an acoustic reflex (contraction of the stapedius muscle) with auditory stimulation also may be obtained with acoustic immittance. Contraction of the stapedius muscle stiffens the TM, increasing its impedance. The reflex arc, which is bilateral, provides information about the status of both middle ears and facial nerves (stapedius muscle). A middle ear effusion prevents meaningful interpretation of an acoustic reflex, since change in impedance relating to the stapedius contraction is insignificant to the change related to a middle ear disorder. Because the acoustic reflex is often absent in neonates and young infants, screening in this patient population is of little use.

Audiometry

Identification of hearing loss in the pediatric population is essential to early habilitation and integration. Hearing impairment associated with OM is most commonly a conductive loss related to an AOM with effusion or a chronic serous/mucoid effusion. A more 'permanent' conductive loss may occur with pathologic changes of the ossicles (erosion or discontinuity) or tympanosclerosis. Some observers believe that a sensorineural loss may occur either temporarily or permanently secondary to in-

Table 3: Auditory Screening*

Neonates

- Family history of sensorineural hearing loss
- In utero infection (eg, cytomegalovirus, syphilis, herpes, toxoplasmosis)
- Craniofacial anomalies/stigmata
- Hyperbilirubinemia
- Ototoxic medication
- Bacterial meningitis
- Low Apgar score
- NICU/ventilation

Infants

- Neurofibromatosis type 2
- Head trauma (fracture or loss of consciousness)
- Stigmata/craniofacial anomaly
- Persistent pulmonary hypertension
- Neurodegenerative disorder
- Parental concern
- Bacterial meningitis
- Recurrent or persistent serous otitis media

* Joint Committee on Infant Hearing: 1994 position statement

creased tension at the round window or to the spread of infection through the round or oval window.

Audiologic referral is recommended in children with speech and language delay, short attention span, familial history of hearing loss, or parental concern of hearing loss.

The 1994 Joint Committee on Infant Hearing position statement identified infants and children for whom auditory screening was recommended (Table 3). Audiologic assessment is important to describe the type (conductive, sensorineural, or mixed), degree, and configuration of the hearing loss. A number of behavioral and nonbehavioral tests are useful for providing such information.

Behavioral testing is the cornerstone of the pediatric audiologic assessment. However, these tests are more subjective and tester dependent compared with nonbehavioral ones. Behavioral testing may be used in infants and children older than 6 months.

The two basic methods for obtaining the data during a behavioral auditory test are conditioned and unconditioned responses. The method selected depends on the age and the cooperation of the child. Conditioned responses rely on rewards provided after each appropriate response to an auditory stimulus. Unconditioned responses require the child to respond voluntarily without providing a reward. Children undergoing unconditioned testing tend to habituate quickly, correlating with their loss of interest.

The most basic qualitative, rather than quantitative, neonatal auditory assessment involves the Moro's and aural-palpebral reflex, during which the baby responds spontaneously to a certain sound pressure level. The next most basic test is behavioral observation audiometry, which is most commonly used in young infants. Simple behavioral responses are observed with auditory stimulants such as rattles and bells. Overt responses include eye movement or head turning; subtle movements include a startle, eye blink, or limb movement.

Visual reinforcement (blinking light) and tangible reinforcement (candy) audiometry are conditioned responses. These reinforcements or rewards are provided when the conditioned child either turns his or her head toward the sound stimulus or presses a bar with stimulus presentation. Studies have shown that 85% to 90% of de-

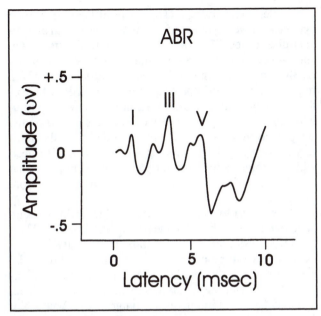

Figure 9: *Auditory brain stem response.*

velopmentally normal 6-month-olds can be accurately tested with visual reinforcement audiometry. While visual reinforcement audiometry is appropriate in infants, preschool children lose interest quickly and require more tangible rewards. Such tests provide information about the level of hearing loss, but do not differentiate between conductive and sensorineural losses.

Conventional audiometry assesses both air and bone conduction with a combination of pure tone and speech audiometry. Similar to adult testing, the child must overtly indicate when the auditory signal is heard. Children older than 5 years are appropriate for conventional audiometry. Play audiometry using games to help determine a threshold is more successful in children 2 and older.

An electrophysiologic assessment of hearing is often necessary in very young infants and in those with significant disabilities. The two most widely used tests are the auditory evoked potentials (or auditory brain stem response [ABR]) and otoacoustic emissions (OAE), neither of which requires the patient's participation. The ABR, which is the most common technique, measures brain waves stimulated by clicks (Figure 9). EEG electrodes placed on the scalp measure a pattern of wave recorded from the auditory nerve along the brain-stem auditory nerve. This test, which eliminates the need for participation, requires that the child be asleep or sedated to avoid interference from muscle activity.

Measuring otoacoustic emissions has recently been developed as an 'objective measurement' to test cochlear activity. Otoacoustic emissions are minute sounds associated with the outer hair cells transmitted from the cochlea through the middle ear and into the external canal. They reflect the functional integrity of the cochlea, and may be found in infants as young as 1 to 2 days old. The role of otoacoustic emissions in pediatric auditory screening is still being investigated.

Selected Readings

1. Joint Committee on Infant Hearing: 1994 position statement. *ASHA* 1994;36:38-41.

2. Lalwani AK, Grundfast KM: *Pediatric Otology and Neurotology*. Philadelphia, Lippincott-Raven, 1998.

3. Potsic WP, Handler SD, Wetmore RF, et al: *Primary Care Pediatric Otolaryngology*. New Jersey, J. Michael Ryan, 1995.

4. Shanks J, Shelton C: Basic principles and clinical applications of tympanometry. *Otolaryngol Clin North Am* 1991;24:299-328.

5. Wilson WR, Richardson MA: Behavioral audiometry. *Otolaryngol Clin North Am* 1991;24:285-297.

6. Lewis N, Dugdale A, Jerger J, et al: Open-ended tympanometric screening: A new concept. *Arch Otolaryngol* 1975;101:722-725.

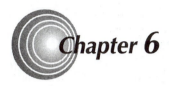

Chapter 6

Antimicrobial Therapy for AOM

Recent changes in susceptibility patterns for organisms that cause acute otitis media (AOM) (Chapter 4) have greatly influenced the approach to first-line therapy, and have modified responses to the recurring question: is amoxicillin at its current dosage recommendation (20 to 40 mg/kg/d) still the drug of choice for AOM?[1] In 2000, more compelling data exist to support consideration of other classes of antibiotics for primary therapy. Macrolides such as azithromycin (Zithromax®) and clarithromycin (Biaxin®); most cephalosporins, particularly parenteral ceftriaxone (Rocephin®), oral cefprozil (Cefzil®), and cefpodoxime proxetil (Vantin®); and loracarbef (Lorabid®) (actually a carbacephem antibiotic) all have activity against penicillin-resistant pneumococci and β-lactamase-producing *Haemophilus influenzae* and *Moraxella catarrhalis*.[2] The newer high-dosage form of amoxicillin/clavulanate (Augmentin®) also covers a higher percentage of amoxicillin-resistant organisms.

Each physician must select first-line therapy for otitis media (OM) based on the regional susceptibility data of bacterial pathogens and, more importantly, on the treatment failure rates of previous regimens (Table 1). Regional differences for these variables make it difficult to offer recommendations that are appropriate for all locations. If a decision is made to change from amoxicillin (or trimethoprim/sulfamethoxazole [TMP/SMX, Bactrim™,

Table 1: Variables in Selecting First-Line Antimicrobial Therapy for AOM[2]

Microbiologic efficacy

- Minimum inhibitory concentration
- % of strains susceptible

Clinical efficacy

- rate of treatment failures

Acceptability of current treatment failures

Adverse reactions

Cost

- actual purchase price
- inclusion of antibiotic on HMO or insurance formularies
- co-pay

Compliance issues

- taste
- dosing interval
- dosing duration

Septra®]) as first-line therapy, many options are available (Figure 1 and Tables 2, 3, and 4). Other considerations for selection might include cost and compliance issues. Compliance is enhanced for antibiotics that are better tasting, dosed once or twice rather than 3 or 4 times a day, and given for shorter durations.[3]

A change to other classes of antibiotics for most outpatient infections also offers the theoretic advantage of reversing the trend to penicillin resistance among these organisms by eliminating the pressure for mutation that

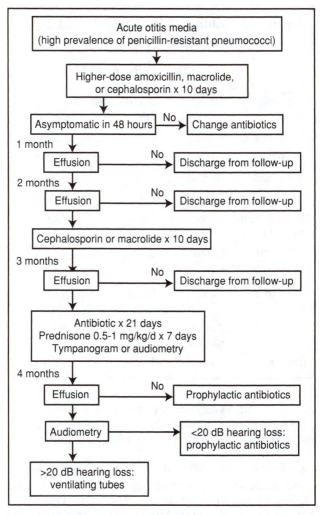

Figure 1: *Algorithm for the management of AOM in geographic regions experiencing a high prevalence of penicillin resistance among clinical isolates of* Streptococcus pneumoniae.

Table 2: Antibiotics for Otitis Media: Cephalosporins

Antibiotic		Daily Dosage/ kg x 10 days	
Generic Name	Trade Name	unless stated otherwise	Interval
ceftriaxone	Rocephin®	50 mg IM	one dose
cefaclor	Ceclor®	40 mg	q 8-12 h
cefadroxil	Duricef®	30 mg	q 12 h
cefixime	Suprax®	8 mg	q 24 h
cefpodoxime proxetil	Vantin®	10 mg	q 12 h
cefprozil	Cefzil®	30 mg	q 12 h
ceftibuten	Cedax®	9 mg	q 24 h
cefuroxime axetil	Ceftin®	30 mg	q 12 h
cephalexin	Keflex®, Keftab®	75 mg	q 6 h
loracarbef	Lorabid®	30 mg	q 12 h

always occurs with excessive use of a single class of agents. Moreover, a change in strategy now may provide the opportunity to return to amoxicillin in the future.

Advantages of Early Antibiotic Treatment

Spontaneous resolution of signs and symptoms after 48 hours occurs in approximately 50% of AOM cases, but this varies significantly by organism. It is lowest for pneumococci (10%), highest for *Moraxella* (70%), and intermediate for *H influenzae* (50%).[4] Because it is impossible to accurately predict which children do not re-

Table 3: Antibiotics for Otitis Media: Macrolides

Antibiotic		Daily Dosage/ kg x 10 days unless stated otherwise	Interval
Generic Name	Trade Name		
azithromycin	Zithromax®	10 mg loading, then 5 mg (4 days)	q 24 h
clarithromycin	Biaxin®	15 mg	q 12 h

quire antibiotics, they should be offered in all cases. Withholding therapy for more than 48 hours, a management option used by some physicians, has been associated with an increase in the incidence of mastoiditis.[5]

Antimicrobial therapy alleviates symptoms within 48 hours in more than 90% of children. Persistence of symptoms after 48 to 72 hours is an indication for empiric change to a different class of antibiotics (Figure 1). In young children, the effusion persists for 1 month in 40% of patients, 2 months in 20%, and 3 months in 10%. Therefore, additional management is not indicated until after 2 months of follow-up for those with persistent effusion, at which time tympanometry should be obtained. Children with a tympanogram showing a C2, C3, or B pattern (Chapter 5), which identifies a growing decrease in compliance of the tympanic membrane, should undergo audiometry. If this testing demonstrates a 20-dB loss or greater, tympanostomy tubes are indicated. This may be necessary in as many as 2% of all AOM cases, representing 10% of all children younger than 3 years.[6]

Table 4: Antibiotics for Otitis Media: Penicillins and Others

Antibiotic		Daily	
Generic Name	Trade Name	Dosage x 10 days	Interval
amoxicillin	Amoxil®, Wymox®	75-90 mg	q 8-12 h
amoxicillin/ clavulanate	Augmentin®	75-90 mg	q 12 h
ampicillin	Omnipen®	50 mg	q 6 h
bacampicillin	Spectrobid®	25-50 mg	q 12 h
clindamycin	Cleocin®	10-20 mg	q 6-8 h
erythromycin/ sulfisoxazole	Pediazole®, Eryzole®	40 mg erythromycin	q 6-8 h
trimethoprim/ sulfamethoxazole	Bactrim™, Septra®	8-12 mg TMP, 40-60 mg SMX	q 12 h
ofloxacin	Floxin® ear drops	AOM with tympanostomy tubes, 5 drops b.i.d. for 10 days; CSOM, 10 drops b.i.d. for 14 days	q 12 h

Eradication of Middle Ear Pathogens

Sterilization of middle ear fluids (MEF) as determined by a repeat tympanocentesis during therapy has been termed the *in vivo sensitivity test*.[7] It is the best documentation of successful clinical response, and is an optimal

Table 5: In Vivo Eradication of AOM Pathogens, 1969-1991[8]

Antibiotic	% of Patients with Eradication of Bacterial Pathogens		
	S pneumoniae	H influenzae	M catarrhalis
amoxicillin	95%	79%	79%
amoxicillin/ clavulanate	97%	81%	93%
TMP/SMX	88%	75%	100%
cefaclor	82%	67%	88%
cefixime	74%	94%	90%
cefprozil	92%	43%	75%
cefuroxime axetil	100%	80%	100%
cefpodoxime proxetil	83%	95%	60%
ceftriaxone	100%	100%	85%
clarithromycin	100%	80%	80%
placebo	11%	48%	70%

criterion to judge the clinical efficacy of antimicrobial agents in treating AOM. Results for 11 such studies conducted between 1969 and 1991 are summarized in Table 5.[8] Data for control children who received placebo in some of the earlier clinical trials offer the most meaningful information on spontaneous resolution of infection. Among a number of published studies that evaluated the natural history of untreated AOM, most have concluded that approximately 50% of all ear infections resolve spontaneously, but that this occurs most frequently with *M catarrhalis* at a rate of 70%, intermediate for *H influenzae* at

Table 6: Penetration of Antimicrobials Into Middle Ear Fluids (MEF)[10]

Drug	Dose	Serum	MEF	MEF/Serum (%)
		Concentration (µg/mL)		
amoxicillin	13.3 mg/kg	11.2	2.8	25
	15 mg/kg	13.6	5.6	41
	1 g	15.3	6.2	41
penicillin V	13.3 mg/kg	8.1	1.8	22
	26 mg/kg	15.5	6.3	41
cefaclor	13.3 mg/kg	3.6	1.0	28
	15 mg/kg	8.5	0.5	6
	15 mg/kg	16.8	3.8	23
	20 mg/kg	29	5.1	18
	40 mg/kg	33	5.9	18
cefuroxime axetil	250 mg	5.4	1.2	22
cefixime	8 mg/kg	2.5	1.3	52
	8 mg/kg	4.2	1.5	36
	5 mg/kg	2.0	0.2	10
cefprozil	15 mg/kg	5.5	2.0	36
	15 mg/kg	12.1	2.0	17
azithromycin	5 mg/kg	1.7	3.6	212

50%, and lowest for *Streptococcus pneumoniae* at only 10%. These data are similar to those in Table 2. Other experiences have varied. One recent study concluded that as many as 80% of patients may not require antimicrobial therapy, the highest reported rate of spontaneous cure.[9]

Pharmacokinetics of Antimicrobials in OME and AOM

Antibiotics penetrate the middle ear mucosa and interstitial fluid through a rich capillary bed and a relatively

Drug	Dose	Concentration (µg/mL)		MEF/ Serum (%)
		Serum	MEF	
loracarbef	7.5 mg/kg	9.3	3.9	42
	9 mg/kg	6.7	9.3	76
trimethoprim	4 mg/kg	2.0	1.4	70
	4 mg/kg	3.1	2.0	65
sulfamethoxazole	20 mg/kg	44.6	8.2	18
	20 mg/kg	70.3	18.7	27
sulfisoxazole	37.5 mg/kg	106	20.9	20
erythromycin ES	12.5 mg/kg	1.0	<0.2	<20
	15 mg/kg	1.2	0.5	42
erythromycin E	15 mg/kg	3.6	1.7	49
clarithromycin	7.5 mg/kg	1.7	2.5	1.47
14-hydroxy-metabolite	0.8	1.3	1.62	

large surface area, producing concentrations in the middle ear that are generally 20% to 50% of those in serum (Table 6).[10] Most of the data summarized in Table 6 were obtained from children with otitis media with effusion (OME) where concentrations of antibiotics may be somewhat lower than those in AOM fluids. The newer macrolides, azithromycin and, to a lesser extent clarithromycin, penetrate into white blood cells, obtaining concentrations that are actually higher than those in serum.

Table 7: Resistant *Streptococcus pneumoniae*—1997 U.S. Surveillance[11]

	% of Isolates		
	Susceptible	Intermediate Resistance	High-Level Resistance
penicillin	56.1	27.8	16.0
azithromycin	85.9	2.4	11.7
clarithromycin	85.6	1.7	12.7
amoxicillin/ clavulanate	80.8	1.1	18.1
amoxicillin	80.7	1.2	18.1
cefpodoxime proxetil	79.1	2.3	18.6
cefuroxime axetil	76.9	3.6	19.5
cefixime	67.0	5.2	27.8
cefaclor	28.5	33.2	38.3
TMP/SMX	74.4	5.8	19.8

A few antibiotics have relatively long serum half-lives that allow for once-a-day dosing. These include azithromycin, the oral cephalosporins cefixime (Suprax®) and ceftibuten (Cedax®), and the parenteral cephalosporin ceftriaxone. Azithromycin, because of its long half-life and accumulation in white blood cells, needs to be given for only 5 days to provide bactericidal activity within the infected middle ear for 10 days. Ceftriaxone retains a level well above the minimum inhibitory concentration (MIC) for common AOM pathogens both in the serum and middle ear for 72 hours or longer, thereby allowing a single dose (50 mg/kg, maximum 1 g) for effective treatment of AOM. This option is preferred for children who are vomiting or for whom compliance with oral antibiotics is a problem.

The gastrointestinal absorption of amoxicillin is quite consistent, even in children with significant diarrhea, and has been shown to be superior to oral ampicillin. Therefore, amoxicillin has replaced ampicillin as the penicillin of choice for common outpatient infections in children. The primary issue for this antibiotic is the dosage required to cover pneumococci during a time of a high degree of penicillin resistance (Tables 6 and 7).[11] The current recommendation is to administer a dosage of 75 to 90 mg/kg/d to achieve middle ear fluid levels of 2 μg/mL or higher to cover more than 90% of *S pneumoniae*. To achieve maximal success, clinicians in Europe have even suggested a dosage of 120 to 150 mg/kg/d.[12]

Pharmacodynamics of Antimicrobials

Because bacterial killing is not enhanced by drug concentrations above the MIC and minimum bactericidal concentration (MBC) for β-lactam antibiotics, investigators have examined other variables that might additionally predict increased efficacy. One important determinant appears to be the percentage of time at the infected tissue site that antibiotic concentrations exceed the MIC of the invading bacterium (Tables 8 and 9). Animal studies have suggested that maximal killing occurs when concentrations of the antibiotic continue for 60% to 70% of the total treatment time, and are generally adequate for AOM when this occurs for only 40% to 50% of the dosing interval. This characteristic of antibiotics is included in the general category of pharmacodynamics. Although data are incomplete, a correlation between time above the MIC in serum and bacteriologic eradication (microbiologic cure) has been supported in retrospective clinical trials of various antibiotics.[10] More than half of the differences in bacteriologic

Table 8: Time Above MIC for Various Antimicrobials Against *S pneumoniae*, *H influenzae*, and *M catarrhalis*[10]

Drug	*S pneumoniae*	
	MIC$_{90}$ (μg/mL)	T>MIC
amoxicillin	0.06	100
plus clavulanate	0.12	100
cefaclor	0.5	44
cefuroxime axetil	0.12	73
cefixime	0.5	48
cefpodoxime proxetil	0.25	62
cefprozil	0.25	78
loracarbef	0.5	42
ceftriaxone	0.06	100
trimethoprim/ sulfamethoxazole	1	100
erythromycin ES	0.06	88
clarithromycin	0.06	100
azithromycin	0.06	100

efficacy may be attributable to this pharmacodynamic variable.

The other more traditional measure that correlates highly with clinical and microbiologic efficacy is the MEF concentration of the antibiotic, particularly how it relates to the MIC of the responsible bacterial pathogen. An analysis of published data indicates that an MEF:MIC ratio above 10 predicts maximal efficacy, while ratios of 3 to 6

H influenzae		M catarrhalis	
MIC_{90}(μg/mL)	T>MIC	MIC_{90}(μg/mL)	T>MIC
1	59	2	46
2	41	0.25	78
8	0	2	35
2	33	2	33
0.06	88	0.5	48
0.12	82	1	37
8	16	2	41
8	9	2	26
0.12	100	0.25	100
0.25	100	0.25	100
8	0	0.12	71
4	0	0.25	100
2	100	0.12	100

correlate with 80% to 85% bacterial eradication. Thus, AOM caused by a pneumococcal strain with an MIC of 1.0 μg/mL (intermediate resistance) may not respond to amoxicillin at a dosage of 40 mg/kg/d, which only achieves average MEF concentrations of 2.8, less than 3-fold the MIC of the organism. The increasing percentage of pneumococcal clinical isolates that exhibit intermediate (MIC 0.1 to 1.0 μg/mL) or high-level (MIC +2 μg/mL) resis-

Table 9: Time Above MIC for Various
β-Lactams Against Intermediate
and Resistant *S pneumoniae*[10]

Drug	Dose
amoxicillin	13.3 mg/kg t.i.d.
cefaclor	13.3 mg/kg t.i.d.
cefixime	8 mg/kg q.d.
cefuroxime axetil	250 mg b.i.d.
loracarbef	15 mg/kg b.i.d.
cefpodoxime	5 mg/kg b.i.d.
cefprozil	15 mg/kg b.i.d.
ceftriaxone	50 mg IM q.d.

tance to penicillin is the reason that many experts recommend higher dosages of amoxicillin (Chapter 4). A dosage of 75 to 90 mg/kg/d provides MEF levels above the MIC of organisms with an MIC of 2 μg/mL or less for more than 40% of the dosing interval, and provides MEF concentrations 10-fold above the MIC for organisms that would be classified as intermediately resistant.[13]

Postantibiotic Effect

Another important pharmacodynamic property in assessing the microbiologic activity of various antimicro-

Penicillin-intermediate *S pneumoniae*		Penicillin-resistant *S pneumoniae*	
MIC_{50-90}	T>MIC	MIC_{50-90}	T>MIC
0.25-1	83-59	1-2	59-46
8-16	0	32-64	0
4-16	0	32-64	0
0.5-2	53-33	4-8	23-0
2-16	26-0	16	0
0.25-2	54-0	2-4	0
0.5-4	66-28	4-16	28-0
0.5	100	1	100

bial agents is the post-MIC effect, commonly termed the postantibiotic effect (PAE). This is defined in an in vitro system where bacteria are exposed to decreasing concentrations of antibiotics that simulate the in vivo kinetics of the specific agents. In the absence of antibiotics, organisms grow rapidly, and the time of replication to a 10-fold ($1 \log_{10}$/mL) increase is determined. The PAE is a measure of the increase in time required for organisms to achieve this 10-fold growth.

The pharmacodynamic properties of the newer macrolides azithromycin and clarithromycin differ some-

Table 10: Adverse Reactions During Antibiotic Treatment for AOM

Antibiotic	Gastrointestinal (%)	Others
amoxicillin	3-18	allergic skin
amoxicillin/ clavulanate	11-33	rash and nonimmunologic rash with Epstein-Barr virus (EBV) infection
cephalosporins	5-15	
cefaclor	10-27	serum sickness
cefixime	18-29	
macrolides	3-6	
TMP/SMX	9-10	Stevens-Johnson syndrome
erythromycin/ sulfisoxazole	13-20	Stevens-Johnson syndrome; increased theophylline concentrations
clindamycin	4-9	pseudo-membranous colitis

what from the β-lactam antibiotics and TMP/SMX in that they exhibit minimal concentration-dependent killing, but a significant postantibiotic effect. However, the main determinant for efficacy of this antibiotic class is still the duration of time that MEF levels exceed the MIC. Macrolides such as azithromycin, with a long serum and tissue half-life, therefore demonstrate more consistent in vivo bactericidal activity. For all macrolides, including erythromycin, the prolonged postantibiotic effect affords higher eradication rates for *S pneumoniae* and *H influenzae*, even when concentrations exceed the MIC of these pathogens for less than 40% of the dosing interval.

Compliance

Several factors influence selection of antimicrobial therapy. Efficacy is certainly the first consideration, yet new antibiotics have rarely demonstrated improved clinical effectiveness over older therapeutic agents. The second factor is comparative toxicity. However, since few marketed antibiotics produce significant adverse reactions, this is rarely an important discriminator (Table 10). The next issues are compliance and cost.

Compliance for completing therapy in young pediatric patients primarily depends on taste of suspension medications. Every parent knows that bitter products result in a daily struggle with their infants. This influences their preferences for therapy to the point that many prefer injectable antibiotics.[3] Therefore, a great deal of effort is expended in improving the palatability of antimicrobial suspension agents.

Table 11 presents taste evaluations for the most commonly prescribed antibiotics for AOM, using amoxicillin as a standard, assigning it a score of 5.0 for comparison to other antibiotics.[3] The overall score category gives extra weight to the ratings for taste and aftertaste. As a group, cephalosporins were ranked higher than other classes, with the exceptions of cefuroxime axetil (Ceftin®) and cefpodoxime proxetil, which were the lowest among these 11 antibiotics.

Adults assume that extremely poor taste jeopardizes children's compliance with medications. Experience in clinical practice supports the importance of taste in medication prescribing for all ages, although judgment of acceptable vs. unacceptable agents is quite variable. On the other hand, some studies have concluded that taste is a

Table 11: Palatability of Antimicrobial Suspensions Commonly Used for AOM[14]

Product	Appearance Mean (SD)	Smell Mean (SD)
1. loracarbef	6.2 (1.9)	6.8 (2.1)
2. cefixime	5.2 (2.0)	5.1 (2.0)
3. azithromycin	6.0 (1.7)	6.3 (1.6)
4. cefprozil	6.4 (2.2)	6.7 (2.1)
5. clarithromycin	5.6 (2.2)	6.4 (2.2)
6. amoxicillin/ clavulanate	5.3 (1.8)	6.0 (2.0)
7. erythromycin/ sulfisoxazole	4.9 (1.9)	6.1 (2.1)
8. trimethoprim/ sulfamethoxazole	5.7 (2.1)	5.3 (2.0)
9. cefuroxime axetil	4.7 (2.0)	5.5 (2.1)
10. cefpodoxime proxetil	4.3 (2.0)	5.0 (2.5)

minor issue in compliance for infants and young children. One study determined that children younger than 6 years old were unable to distinguish taste differences between formulations. More recent evaluations, however, did not find differences based on age, concluding that the sense of taste is well developed in early infancy, with the only variation being a waning with advanced age.

Categories			
Texture Mean (SD)	Taste Mean (SD)	Aftertaste Mean (SD)	Average overall score
6.5 (2.1)	7.4 (2.1)	7.0 (2.4)	7.0
5.9 (1.8)	5.4 (2.3)	6.0 (2.0)	5.5
5.0 (1.6)	5.5 (2.1)	3.5 (2.3)	5.1
5.5 (1.6)	4.1 (2.1)	4.6 (2.6)	5.0
3.5 (2.0)	5.4 (2.3)	3.3 (2.4)	4.8
4.9 (1.8)	3.8 (1.9)	4.2 (2.1)	4.5
4.5 (2.1)	3.4 (2.0)	3.7 (1.9)	4.1
5.3 (1.7)	3.1 (2.0)	2.1 (2.0)	3.7
3.0 (2.0)	1.7 (1.4)	1.3 (1.1)	2.6
3.7 (2.2)	1.8 (1.7)	1.2 (1.1)	2.6

Other considerations for selection include cost. With current dosing recommendations, only one antibiotic, TMP/SMX, is considered inexpensive, ie, less than $20 for a 10-day course for a 13-kg 2-year-old (Table 12). Those costing $20 to $40 are clarithromycin, amoxicillin, and erythromycin/sulfisoxazole; more expensive at $40 to $60 are loracarbef, azithromycin (5-day course),

Table 12: Cost of Commonly Used Antibiotic Suspensions (1999)*

Generic name Flavor	Trade name Cost*	Manufacturer
trimethoprim/ sulfamethoxazole cherry	Bactrim™ $9.75	Roche
clarithromycin fruit punch	Biaxin® $19.86	Abbott
amoxicillin strawberry	Amoxil® $31.80	SmithKline Beecham
erythromycin/ sulfisoxazole strawberry/banana	Pediazole® $38.40	Ross

loracarbef
  strawberry
  bubble gum
	Lorabid®
	$46.18
		Lilly

azithromycin cherry	Zithromax® $49.00	Pfizer
cefuroxime axetil tutti-frutti	Ceftin® $53.39	Glaxo Wellcome
cefprozil bubble gum	Cefzil® $58.66	Bristol-Myers Squibb
amoxicillin/ clavulanate banana	Augmentin® $74.51	SmithKline Beecham
cefixime strawberry	Suprax® $76.24	Lederle
cefpodoxime proxetil lemon creme	Vantin® $133.95	Pharmacia & Upjohn

* Based on a survey of 5 drugstore chains in New Orleans, La. *Infect Med* 1999;16:197-200.

cefuroxime axetil, and cefprozil; and most costly (>$70) are amoxicillin/clavulanate, cefixime, and cefpodoxime proxetil.

Pollyanna Phenomenon

Perceived clinical responses despite documented bacteriologic failure has been termed the Pollyanna phenomenon, after the young girl in the movie of the same name who saw good in everyone and everything. When tympanocenteses have documented sterilization of MEF, clinical responses were observed in more than 90% of patients. However, bacteriologic failures were judged to be clinical cures in more than half of children enrolled in one large collaborative therapeutic trial.[15]

References

1. Steele RW, Warrier R, Unkel PJ, et al: Colonization with antibiotic-resistant *Streptococcus pneumoniae* in children with sickle cell disease. *J Pediatr* 1996;128:531-535.

2. Steele RW: Management of otitis media. *Infect Med* 1998; 15:174-178, 203.

3. Steele RW, Estrada B, Begue RE, et al: A double-blind taste comparison of pediatric antibiotic suspensions. *Clin Pediatr (Phila)* 1997;36:193-199.

4. Howie VM: Eradication of bacterial pathogens from middle ear infections. *Clin Infect Dis* 1992;14:209-210.

5. Hoppe JE, Koster S, Bootz F, et al: Acute mastoiditis—relevant once again. *Infection* 1994;22:178-182.

6. Kleinman LC, Kosecoff J, Dubois RW, et al: The medical appropriateness of tympanostomy tubes proposed for children younger than 16 years in the United States. *JAMA* 1994;271:1250-1255.

7. Howie VM, Ploussard JH: The "in vivo sensitivity test"—bacteriology of middle ear exudate, during antimicrobial therapy in otitis media. *Pediatrics* 1969;44:940-944.

8. Klein JO: Microbiologic efficacy of antibacterial drugs for acute otitis media. *Pediatr Infect Dis J* 1993;12:973-975.

9. Rosenfeld RM, Vertrees JE, Carr J, et al: Clinical efficacy of antimicrobial drugs for acute otitis media: metaanalysis of 5400

children from thirty-three randomized trials. *J Pediatr* 1994;124: 355-367.

10. Craig WA, Andes D: Pharmacokinetics and pharmacodynamics of antibiotics in otitis media. *Pediatr Infect Dis J* 1996;15: 255-259.

11. Doern GV, Pfaller MA, Kugler K, et al: Prevalence of antimicrobial resistance among respiratory tract isolates of *Streptococcus pneumoniae* in North America: 1997 results from the SENTRY antimicrobial surveillance program. *Clin Infect Dis* 1998;27:764-770.

12. Roger G, Carles P, Pangon B, et al: Management of acute otitis media caused by resistant pneumococci in infants. *Pediatr Infect Dis J* 1998;17:631-638.

13. Canafax DM, Yuan Z, Chonmaitree T, et al: Amoxicillin middle ear fluid penetration and pharmacokinetics in children with acute otitis media. *Pediatr Infect Dis J* 1998;17:149-156.

14. Bauchner H, Adams W, Barnett E, et al: Therapy for acute otitis media. Preference of parents for oral or parenteral antibiotic. *Arch Pediatr Adolesc Med* 1996;150:396-399.

15. Marchant CD, Carlin SA, Johnson CE, et al: Measuring the comparative efficacy of antibacterial agents for otitis media: the "Pollyanna phenomenon". *J Pediatr* 1992;120:72-77.

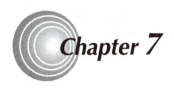

Chapter 7

Withholding Antibiotics, Short-Course Therapy, and Delayed Therapy

F ew treatments are more time-honored than early institution of antibiotics for acute otitis media (AOM) in children. Few current texts, antibiotic treatment manuals, or review articles recommend delaying or withholding antimicrobial therapy for documented ear infections.

Why should we challenge this prevailing dogma? Articles have only recently appeared in the American[1,2] and European medical literature[3-6] suggesting that fewer children should be treated with antibiotics for AOM. The primary reason for this change is the worldwide decrease in susceptibility of bacteria to many classes of antimicrobial agents, resulting in higher morbidity and overall medical costs. Resistance has been reported for the three most common bacterial causes of otitis media (OM). Intermediate and high-level resistance of pneumococci to penicillin approaches 50%, and is attributable to a change in penicillin-binding proteins, while β-lactamase production by *Haemophilus influenzae* is 50% and by *Moraxella catarrhalis* is 100% throughout the United States and in many European countries.

Shortly after the introduction of antibiotics for routine therapy of AOM, the overall incidence of mastoiditis and otitic meningitis decreased significantly, although no particular clinical study proved that early antimicrobial therapy was responsible for this change.[3] Despite the absence of supportive data, prevention of suppurative sequelae was attributed to the early eradication of middle ear pathogens. Unfortunately, it still remains uncertain whether the decline of mastoiditis and meningitis during the 1950s resulted from antimicrobial therapy or from changes in the clinical course, organism virulence, or increased host resistance. Also, some have postulated that routine cases of uncomplicated OM did not attract medical attention during the preantibiotic era, thereby yielding the appearance that the overall rate of suppurative complications was high.

In addition to prevention of disease extension, another argument for aggressive treatment of OM is to eliminate middle ear effusion and reverse the hearing loss associated with infection. This issue is reviewed extensively in Chapter 3. Some clinicians also believe that antibiotics provide more rapid bacteriologic and clinical resolution, as well as prevent recurrent infection.

The European Experience

In many countries in Europe, particularly the Netherlands, the United Kingdom, and Germany, selective use of antimicrobials has become increasingly popular. Surveys have indicated that the routine use of antibiotics for AOM is lowest in the Netherlands, at just 31% of doctors monitored, while in the United States and Australia virtually 100% of physicians treat all diagnosed cases with antibiotics.[3]

Why such a difference in the Netherlands? In 1990, the Dutch College of Family Doctors published guidelines on the management of AOM[3] (Table 1). This strategy emphasized symptomatic treatment with antipyretics and decongestants for the first 3 days in children as young as 6 months. The patient was reevaluated if symptoms persisted for 3 days or longer in children 2 years of age or

Table 1: Dutch Guidelines for the Treatment of Acute Otitis Media[6]

Patients 2 years and older

- Treatment of symptoms only (paracetamol with or without decongestant nose drops) for the first 3 days.

- Reevaluation if symptoms (pain or fever thought to be caused by AOM) continue for 3 days. At that time, the physician may continue additional observation or give an antimicrobial (amoxicillin, or erythromycin if amoxicillin is contraindicated) for 7 days.

- Special treatment for tympanic membrane perforation is not suggested unless it persists for 14 days, at which time a course of antimicrobials is suggested.

Children between ages 6 months and 2 years

- Management is the same as those for 2 years and older, except for a mandatory contact (either telephone or visit) after 24 hours. If there is no improvement, physicians may either start antimicrobials or wait an additional 24 hours.

- Referral to an otolaryngologist suggested if patients in this age group appear seriously ill or do not improve after 24 hours of treatment with antimicrobials.

older, but mandatory reexamination 1 day after diagnosis was recommended for children younger than 2. This approach had been validated by a study published 5 years earlier, in which 4,860 consecutive patients with AOM were managed without antimicrobial therapy.[7] Approxi-

Table 2: Antibiotics in the Treatment of AOM: Placebo-Controlled Clinical Trials

Reference/Year; Population	Outcome
Halsted C, et al: 1968[8] American, 2 to 66 months	Pain at 2 to 7 days: no difference
van Buchem FL, et al: 1981[9] Dutch, 2 to 12 years	Pain at 24 hours: no difference Pain at 2 to 7 days: no difference Recurrent AOM: reduced
Mygind N, et al: 1981[10] Danish, 1 to 10 years	Pain at 2 to 7 days: markedly reduced Perforation: reduced Vomiting, diarrhea, rash: increased Hearing loss: no difference Contralateral AOM: markedly reduced Recurrent AOM: no difference

mately 3% were still moderately ill after 3 to 4 days or had otorrhea for more than 14 days, the definition of severe disease in this study. Only two developed mastoiditis, and both responded to oral antimicrobial therapy. The investigators concluded that selective use of antimicrobials offered the same benefit as routine treatment. This, and the continued experience in the Netherlands, suggest that routine treatment and antimicrobial treatment are equally effective in preventing the complications of mastoiditis and meningitis.

Reference/Year; Population	Outcome

Thalin A, et al: 1985[11]
Swedish, 2 to 15 years
	Pain at 24 hours: no difference
	Pain at 2 to 7 days: reduced
	Vomiting, diarrhea, rash:
	  no difference
	Contralateral AOM:
	  markedly reduced
	Recurrent AOM: no difference

Kaleida PH, et al: 1991[12] American, 7 months to 12 years	Pain at 2 to 7 days: reduced Recurrent AOM: no difference

Burke P, et al: 1991[13]
English, 3 to 10 years
	Pain at 24 hours: no difference
	Pain at 2 to 7 days: reduced
	Perforation: markedly reduced
	Vomiting, diarrhea, rash:
	  increased
	Hearing loss: reduced
	Contralateral AOM:
	  no difference

An older review of publications on the medical management of OM concluded that only 1 of 7 children treated with antibiotics benefited. However, only 4 of the 33 published studies in this analysis included control patients who did not receive antibiotics.[14] A similar review of clinical trials in 50 publications judged that most of these investigations had methodology flaws that prevented adequate evaluation[15]; no conclusion was reached.

A more recent meta-analysis limited to six randomized, placebo-controlled AOM treatment trials in Europe

Table 3: Antibiotic Therapy of AOM in Infants and Children[12]

	Nonsevere		Severe	
	Placebo	Amoxi-cillin	Myringo-tomy	Amoxi-cillin
Pain/fever-free after 24 to 48 hours	92%	96%	76%	90%
Effusion-free at 6 weeks	48%	54%	65%	44%
No recurrence within 6 weeks	72%	72%	83%	59%

and the United States found no difference in the percentage of children who had pain 24 hours after starting antibiotic treatment vs controls, but that the antibiotic group experienced significant reduction of pain 2 to 7 days after beginning therapy (9.7% vs 14.3%).[4] Also, the risk of progression to bilateral OM was reduced by 43% in the treatment group. No differences were found in the incidence of significant hearing loss at 1 month, or in the incidence of recurrent OM. The authors concluded from these studies[8-13] that early use of antibiotics provided clinical advantages, but these were limited to perhaps only 1 in 17 treated children (Table 2). The shortcoming of this meta-analysis is the small number of patients included in individual studies. Once specific outcomes were analyzed, numbers were even more limited, making meaningful comparisons difficult. For example, just a few children experienced perforation of the eardrum or hearing loss after 3 months; thus, differences in the treatment group vs placebo controls of 50% and 20%, respectively, did not achieve statistical significance. More importantly, the

Table 4: Placebo vs Amoxicillin Therapy in Older Children (>3 years), United Kingdom, 1986-1989[13]

	Placebo	Amoxicillin
Fever-free after 24 hours	80%	92%
Pain-free after 6 days	75%	82%
Clinical resolution at 8 days on original treatment	86%	98%
Effusion-free at 1 month	65%	63%
Effusion-free at 3 months	72%	82%
Normal without otolaryngologic referral, by 1 year	92%	94%

incidence of mastoiditis and meningitis was so low that these trials did not even try to analyze the effect of early treatment on these rare complications.

A prospective comparative trial conducted in Pittsburgh from 1981 to 1985 compared placebo to amoxicillin for nonsevere AOM, and myringotomy to amoxicillin for more severe cases[12] (Table 3). Nonsevere was defined as a rectal temperature below 39.5°C and otalgia for less than 12 hours, while severe was defined as rectal temperature above 39.5°C or otalgia for more than 12 hours. This and other studies suggested that the benefits of antibiotic therapy were relatively modest. A similar study conducted in the United Kingdom (Table 4) found neither a difference in pain at 24 hours, nor an increased incidence of contralateral AOM.[13] Benefit, however, was shown for three parameters: pain at 2 to 7 days, a reduction in the incidence of tympanic membrane perforation, and a reduction in overall hearing loss for antibiotics compared with no antibiotics.

Despite these recent studies, primary care physicians in the United Kingdom continue to treat AOM with antibiotics. Most feel that additional data are necessary before risking an increase in suppurative sequelae from delaying or withholding antibiotics. Additional large clinical trials are needed to determine if antibiotics are ineffective in reducing complications of AOM. On the other hand, more judicious use of antibiotics is warranted for children in whom the diagnosis is in doubt, or who tolerate mild infection well enough so that quality of life is not compromised. Withholding antibiotics in these children is reasonable, but only if parents are thoroughly counseled and concur with this approach.

Short-Course Antimicrobial Therapy

A number of therapeutic trials, most conducted in Europe, have examined shorter courses of antimicrobial therapy, from 2 to 7 days, compared to the present standard 10 days' duration. Results have often been equivalent.[1] Many of these studies are difficult to interpret for application in the United States because the antibiotics used and the supportive measures are much different from American standards. Most of these trials examined only children older than 3 years, implying that a departure in therapy might be detrimental to younger children. These trials, however, used antibiotics with short half-lives so that results clearly evaluated duration of therapy as a variable in clinical efficacy. This should not be confused with azithromycin (Zithromax®), which is normally given for only 5 days but, with its long cumulative half-life, remains at concentrations above the minimum inhibitory concentration (MIC) of most AOM pathogens for 10 days or longer.

The most quoted American studies examined 10 days versus 5 days of therapy for cefaclor (Ceclor®)[16] and amoxicillin/clavulanate (Augmentin®).[17] Both studies were double blind and included relatively large numbers of patients. The cefaclor trial enrolled 175 patients with AOM randomized into 10 days of therapy with cefaclor, or 5 days of therapy followed by 5 days of placebo. The dosage of cefaclor was 40 mg/kg/d administered in equally divided doses at 12-hour intervals. Tympanocenteses before treatment were positive in 76% of study patients. *Streptococcus pneumoniae* was recovered in 35% of middle ear specimens, *H influenzae* in 28%, and *M catarrhalis* in 21%. Mixed infections were seen in some of these ear fluids. Treatment failures were found in 10% of patients with 5 days of therapy, and in 6% with 10 days of therapy, a difference that was not significant. Rates of reinfection and persistent middle ear effusion at 10, 30, 60, and 90 days follow-up were not significantly different in the two regimens. This study concluded that patients with AOM and intact tympanic membranes may be treated with the short course (5 days) of cefaclor. One group excluded from this recommendation was children with AOM and with spontaneous purulent drainage. These patients require a longer duration of therapy. The failure rates for this patient population, 53% with 5 days of therapy, versus 8% for 10 days of therapy, were significant, thereby supporting longer duration of treatment.

A more recent study examined 5-day versus 10-day therapy with amoxicillin/clavulanate, although this study was actually designed to validate a new formulation of this product and its administration twice daily (b.i.d.) rather than 3 times daily (t.i.d.). Since the b.i.d. group was divided into short-course and long-course therapy, the two groups could be compared. This study included 868 children with AOM, ages 2 months to 12 years, and the criteria to diagnose AOM and to determine cure and improvement rates were stringent. Treatment successes, categorized as either clinical cure or improvement, occurred in 86.5% (154 of 178) in the 10-day group and

71.1% (140 of 197) in the 5-day group. Corresponding values on days 32 to 38 of follow-up were 63.1% and 57.8%. The 10-day regimen was significantly more effective than the 5-day regimen in younger subjects. The study concluded that administration for 5 days appeared inferior for younger children, but was probably equivalent for patients 6 to 12 years old. The authors recommended that courses shorter than 10 days might be reasonable for AOM in children ages 6 years and older.

Perhaps the best example of success with short-course therapy is clinical results with a single intramuscular dose of ceftriaxone (Rocephin®). Although its serum half-life in children is 6 to 8 hours, serum concentrations above the MIC are unlikely after 3 to 5 days. In comparative clinical trials, this single-dose therapy was as effective as a 10-day course of either amoxicillin or trimethoprim/sulfamethoxazole (TMP/SMX, Bactrim™, Septra®).[18]

Despite a paucity of firm data to adequately evaluate short-course therapy, the expert group assembled by the editors of the journal *Pediatrics* recommended that "uncomplicated AOM may be treated with a 5-to-7 day course of antimicrobials in certain patients," identified only as older children with mild AOM. "Older" was defined as children over 15 months to 2 years. Further discussion by this committee suggested restriction of short-course therapy to children older than 2 years. The reason for this age difference was the limited data on short-course therapy in young children, particularly those with severe or complicated AOM. Most published trials actually excluded young children from short-course therapy because of the known higher incidence of treatment failure and subsequent chronic or recurrent OM.

Complicated courses are more common in the very young, although researchers have speculated that prolonged illnesses in infants are related to concomitant viral infections. Likewise, longer-duration therapy has seemed necessary for children with a perforated tympanic membrane.

The obvious advantage of decreasing therapy of AOM from the traditional 10-day course of antimicrobials is a reduction in total exposure to antibiotics. This is one way of combating the pressure of frequent and prolonged antibiotic use, which has been shown to increase antimicrobial resistance of microorganisms, not only for the individual patient but for the community at large. Particularly pertinent is the observation in day-care centers that the total exposure to antibiotics influences the susceptibility pattern for colonizing bacteria of all children in these centers. The normal behavior of toddlers is such that bacteria are rapidly transferred from one child to another, and these organisms are more likely to be resistant to antimicrobial agents if children have recently been treated for AOM or for other presumed bacterial infections.

Short-course therapy is also supported by compliance studies indicating that, on average, children receive antibiotics for 5 to 7 days regardless of the prescribed duration. Also, the average number of doses received each day is 2, although the prescribed intervals may be 3 or even 4 times a day.

Short-course therapy should be considered with caution because clinical trials comparing 10 days to 5 days of therapy with approved antibiotics have indicated that the longer therapy is superior. These trials have never been published by the companies that conducted them because data did not support a change in prescribing standards.

Delayed Therapy

Another option preferred by some European physicians, and a small number of American physicians, is delayed therapy.[19] With this strategy, once AOM is diagnosed, a prescription for antibiotics is written, but parents are instructed not to fill the prescription unless symptoms persist for more than 48 hours, or worsen during the 2 days after diagnosis. This approach takes advantage of the opportunity to withhold antibiotics from the 40% to 80% of

Table 5: Antibiotics and AOM Recurrences[20]

Antibiotics Initiated	1-Month Recurrence	Any Recurrence
At onset	14%	45%
Day 2 to 7	11%	41%
Day 8 or later	6%	34%
No antibiotic	5%	32%

children whose middle ear infection will resolve spontaneously. Unfortunately, it is impossible to identify these patients during initial evaluation. One study, which included 2,145 children seen in a Danish otolaryngologic clinic setting from 1950 to 1964, suggested that deferring antibiotics for a few days might actually result in better long-term results[20] (Table 5). The authors suggested that this delay permitted children to develop antibodies or other host responses against the invading pathogen, thereby preventing subsequent recurrence of infection. Parents obviously play a significant role in delayed antimicrobial therapy, both in agreeing to deny immediate antimicrobial therapy for their children and in assessing whether symptoms have worsened or have not adequately resolved within 48 hours.

Most experience with this option comes from the Netherlands, where more than two thirds of primary care physicians do not routinely prescribe antibiotics for initial management. Dutch physicians differ about how long to withhold antibiotics, based partly on the child's age and the duration or severity of symptoms. However, the overall experience has supported delayed therapy and has resulted in a slowing of emerging antibiotic resistance in this country.

American physicians have extensively debated the merits of delaying therapy to better control and reduce the total consumption of antibiotics in the United States. The primary rebuttal is that pain, fever, and other symptoms are likely to be prolonged in the 20% to 60% of children who ultimately require antimicrobial therapy. Also, parents' return to work would be delayed, a financial burden for a single parent or for both parents who must work to support the family. Of more concern is the potential for an increase in the incidence of mastoiditis and perhaps otitic meningitis. Further European experience will likely resolve this question.

Are American parents likely to accept delayed therapy once they are counseled on all related issues? The public has been well apprised about the urgent problem of common bacterial resistance to amoxicillin and other first- and second-line antibiotics now used to treat AOM, other outpatient infections, and more importantly, life-threatening infectious processes. Most primary care clinicians, however, have already concluded that parents would insist on early intervention, because physicians for some time have emphasized the detrimental outcomes of delayed diagnosis and management for virtually all infectious diseases. For decades now, we have worked to improve access to medical care, to ensure that all children receive recommended vaccines or other preventive interventions, and to provide optimal medications as rapidly as possible. Supportive care for a documented bacterial infection would represent a marked change in philosophy for both physicians and parents. However, change should be driven by scientific data, and some now exist for delayed antimicrobial therapy of AOM.

References

1.   Dowell SF, Marcy SM, Phillips WR, et al: Otitis media—principles of judicious use of antimicrobial agents. *Pediatrics* 1998;101:165-171.

2.   Bauchner H, Philipp B: Reducing inappropriate oral antibiotic use: a prescription for change. *Pediatrics* 1998;102:142-145.

3.   Froom J, Culpepper L, Jacobs M, et al: Antimicrobials for acute otitis media? A review from the International Primary Care Network. *BMJ* 1997;315:98-102.

4.   Del Mar C, Glasziou P, Hayem M: Are antibiotics indicated as initial treatment for children with acute otitis media? A meta-analysis. *BMJ* 1997;314:1526-1529.

5.   Majeed A, Harris T: Acute otitis media in children. *BMJ* 1997;315:321-322.

6.   Appelman CL, Bossen PC, Dunk JH, et al: Guideline: Acute otitis media. Utrecht, Dutch College of Family Doctors, 1990.

7.   van Buchem FL: Antibiotics for otitis media. *J R Coll Gen Pract* 1987;37:367.

8.   Halsted C, Lepow ML, Balassanian N, et al: Otitis media. Clinical observations, microbiology, and evaluation of therapy. *Am J Dis Child* 1968;115:542-551.

9.   van Buchem FL, Dunk JH, van't Hof MA: Therapy of acute otitis media: myringotomy, antibiotics, or neither? A double-blind study in children. *Lancet* 1981;2:883-887.

10. Mygind N, Meistrup-Larsen KI, Thomsen J, et al: Penicillin in acute otitis media: a double-blind placebo-controlled trial. *Clin Otolaryngol* 1981;6:5-13.

11. Thalin A, Densert O, Larrson A, et al: Is penicillin necessary in the treatment of acute otitis media? In: *Proceedings of the International Conference on Acute and Secretory Otitis Media*, Part 1. Jerusalem, Israel, November 17-22. Amsterdam, Kugler Publications, 1985, pp 441-446.

12. Kaleida PH, Casselbrant ML, Rockette HE, et al: Amoxicillin or myringotomy or both for acute otitis media: results of a randomized clinical trial. *Pediatrics* 1991;87:466-474.

13. Burke P, Bain J, Robinson D, et al: Acute red ear in children: controlled trial of non-antibiotic treatment in general practice. *BMJ* 1991;303:558-562.

14. Rosenfeld RM, Vertrees JE, Carr J, et al: Clinical efficacy of antimicrobial drugs for acute otitis media: metaanalysis of 5400 children from thirty-three randomized trials. *J Pediatr* 1994; 124:355-367.

15. Claessen JQ, Appelman CL, Touw-Otten FW, et al: A review of clinical trials regarding treatment of acute otitis media. *Clin Otolaryngol* 1992;17:251-257.

16. Hendrickse WA, Kusmiesz H, Shelton S, et al: Five vs. ten days of therapy for acute otitis media. *Pediatr Infect Dis J* 1988; 7:14-23.

17. Hoberman A, Paradise JL, Burch DJ, et al: Equivalent efficacy and reduced occurrence of diarrhea from a new formulation of amoxicillin/clavulanate potassium (Augmentin) for treatment of acute otitis media in children. *Pediatr Infect Dis J* 1997;16: 463-470.

18. Dowell SF, Butler JC, Giebink GS, et al: Acute otitis media: management and surveillance in an era of pneumococcal resistance—a report from the Drug-Resistant *Streptococcus pneumoniae* Therapeutic Working Group. *Pediatr Infect Dis J* 1999;18:1-9.

19. Cunningham AS: Antibiotics for otitis media: restraint, not routine. *Contemp Pediatr* 1994;11:17-30.

20. Diamant M, Diamant B: Abuse and timing of use of antibiotics in acute otitis media. *Arch Otolaryngol* 1974;100:226-232.

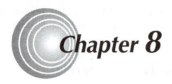

Chapter 8

Adjunctive Therapy

B ecause the main objectives in managing acute otitis
media (AOM) and otitis media with effusion (OME)
are sterilization along with subsequent elimination
of middle ear fluid, a number of clinical studies have combined antibiotics with options that might enhance drainage of middle ear effusions. These adjunctive approaches
have included both medical and surgical interventions
(Table 1). Most of the studies examining topical and oral
decongestants and oral antihistamines were conducted in
the 1960s and 1970s. Surgical adjunctive therapy was studied somewhat later. Few data are available from clinical
trials conducted in the 1990s, and additional studies are
unlikely to be performed, even though the methodology
and study design of earlier reports were often flawed.
Exceptions are current trials designed to examine the benefits of early tympanostomy tube placement on speech
development and cognitive function in children with
chronic OME.

Both topical and systemic decongestants remain the
most popular among pediatricians in managing uncomplicated AOM and OME. Earlier surgical interventions
are likely for more recalcitrant or complicated patients.
The medical options are directed at opening the eustachian tubes by drying secretions, as well as the mucosa
and adenoid tissue at the outlet of the eustachian tube.
Surgical procedures provide drainage through the tympanic membrane after myringotomy or placement of
tympanostomy tubes. Tonsillectomy and adenoidectomy

Table 1: Potential Adjunctive Therapy for AOM and OME

- Topical decongestants
- Oral decongestants
- Antihistamines
- Corticosteroids
- Allergy control
- Myringotomy
- Adenoidectomy
- Tympanostomy tubes

have been examined as methods of reducing congested tissue at the outlet of the eustachian tube when decongestants or antihistamines fail. Researchers have long believed that allergy is involved in the slow resolution of middle ear fluid, particularly in children with asthma or other documented allergic diatheses, children with strong family histories of allergic disease, and patients who have signs and symptoms suggestive of respiratory allergy at the time they are diagnosed with AOM or OME.

Although it may seem rational to offer methods of potentially increasing drainage of middle ear fluid, virtually all approaches, both medical and surgical, have remained controversial because well-designed studies have generally shown variable benefit. On the other hand, most adjunctive options are supported by one or more trials. Although some children might benefit from combination therapy, most are unlikely to have an improved outcome.

Topical Decongestants

Nose drops and nasal sprays are the simplest and most direct approaches to decongestion of the mucosa of the

Table 2: Topical Nasal Decongestants for AOM and OME: Placebo-Controlled Trials

Topical decongestant	Results	Reference
Phenylephrine nasal spray	No improvement in otologic status	Collipp (1961)[1]
Ephedrine nose drops	No improvement in audiometric findings or tympanic membrane compliance	Fraser et al (1977)[2]
Ephedrine nasal spray	No effect on eustachian tube function or resolution of AOM	Cantekin et al (1980)[3]
Oxymetazoline nasal spray	No effect on eustachian tube function or resolution of AOM	Lildholdt et al (1982)[4]
Beclomethasone nasal spray	Effective in only 3 of 10 children with OME	Schwartz et al (1980)[5]
Beclomethasone nasal spray	No efficacy observed for OME	Lildholdt et al (1982)[4]

eustachian tube and structures near its outlet. Theoretically, decongestion allows for drainage of middle ear fluid into the posterior oropharynx, and reverses the negative

pressure in the middle ear cavity, which promotes accumulation of serous fluid. A number of studies have at-
tempted to document clinical efficacy, usually when topical decongestants were used in conjunction with antibiotics
in the early management of AOM[1-4] or used alone for the
treatment of OME[4,5] (Table 2). None has clearly supported
the addition of topical decongestant therapy in the treatment of AOM or OME.

A typical study of the 1960s was one by Collipp,[1]
which included 180 children with AOM. Half received
phenylephrine hydrochloride nose drops along with penicillin and sulfisoxazole. An oral antihistamine, chlorpheniramine maleate, and an oral decongestant, phenylephrine hydrochloride, were also given to all participants.
No differences were noted in the appearance of the tympanic membrane, resolution of middle ear fluid, or in
the rapidity of disappearance of clinical symptoms for
those who received nose drops. A study conducted by
Fraser et al[2] in the 1970s compared ephedrine nose drops
to no treatment for children with OME. No difference in
audiometric parameters was observed. A significant
problem in this study was that various combinations of
oral antihistamines and decongestants, as well as
autoinflation, were examined in some groups, making it
difficult to clearly evaluate the contributions of topical
decongestant therapy.

A more recent study[4] examined potential benefits of
oxymetazoline hydrochloride nasal spray in the management of both AOM and OME in children. The 40 study
participants all had tympanostomy tubes, which allowed
for assessment of tubal function before and after spraying the nose with the nasal spray or placebo. No benefits
were demonstrated.

The conclusion of the Otitis Media Guideline Panel
for the management of OME[6] (Chapter 11) indirectly dis-
couraged the use of topical decongestants, based on a
lack of clear documentation for efficacy.

Table 3: Oral Decongestants and Antihistamines for AOM and OME: Placebo-Controlled Trials

Decongestant/ Antihistamine	Results	Reference
Pseudoephedrine	No improvement in resolution of AOM	Rubenstein et al (1965)[7]
Carbinoxamine plus pseudoephedrine	Children with tympanostomy tubes and effusion: improvement of eustachian tube function in 6 of 13	Miller (1970)[8]
Chlorpheniramine	More rapid response and improved outcome	Stickler et al (1967)[9]
Pseudoephedrine	No benefit	Olson et al (1978)[10]
Ephedrine plus chlorpheniramine	Improved eustachian tube function in 40% of treated patients	Holmquist (1977)[11]

Oral Decongestants and Antihistamines

Studies examining oral decongestants with or without antihistamines for OME have been somewhat more promising than those evaluating topical decongestants, although study design has often not been adequate for meaningful interpretation[2,3,7-13] (Table 3). Most importantly, these early clinical trials included large numbers of study patients with

Decongestant/ Antihistamine	Results	Reference
Brompheniramine plus phenylephrine plus phenylpropanolamine	No benefit	Fraser et al (1977)[2]
Pseudoephedrine	Improvement in eustachian tube function	Cantekin et al (1980)[3]
Pseudoephedrine plus chlorpheniramine	No efficacy for OME	Cantekin et al (1983)[12]
Decongestant and antihistamine	No benefit	Mandel (1987)[13]

fairly well-defined disease. Some concluded that systemic decongestant therapy was as effective as adjunctive treatment,[3,8,9,11] while others failed to show benefit.[2,7,10,12,13]

Some studies included tympanometry and other measurements of eustachian tube function,[3,8,11] and all showed at least some improvement of mechanisms, which should allow for increased drainage of middle ear fluid. Most used a combination of an oral decongestant and antihistamine. One report examined 13 children with tympanostomy tubes and effusion.[8] Improvement of eustachian tube function occurred in 6 who were treated with combination decongestant/antihistamine medications. The number of children included was small, but the study still points out that benefits are quite variable. As in many other medical therapies, treatment should be discontinued in patients who show no response.

One placebo-controlled trial conducted by Cantekin et al[3] included 22 children with upper respiratory infections and altered eustachian tube function. An oral decongestant, pseudoephedrine hydrochloride, significantly improved function by the second day of therapy. In a subsequent study of 28 children with abnormal eustachian tube function but without respiratory disease, these investigators also found that combination decongestant plus antihistamine therapy produced the same benefits. However, they subsequently conducted a double-blind, placebo-controlled trial that included 553 children with OME, and were unable to demonstrate clinical efficacy.[12] This excellent study is the primary basis for the conclusion of the Otitis Media Guideline Panel on the management of OME: "Antihistamine/decongestant therapy is not recommended for treatment of otitis media with effusion in a child of any age, because review of the literature showed that these agents are not effective for this condition, either separately or together."

Only one large randomized trial of AOM demonstrated efficacy for the addition of an oral antihistamine as adjunctive therapy.[9] This study compared penicillin alone to combination penicillin plus chlorpheniramine maleate. The combination group had more rapid resolution of symptoms along with a higher clinical cure rate. Not all children had middle ear effusions, which is now required to make a diagnosis of AOM. An additional problem with this study, as well as with others that have examined antihistamines, is the common excessive drowsiness and irritability that result from these medications.

Thus, too few data support the routine addition of oral decongestants or antihistamines in the management of OME or AOM. On the other hand, in the Netherlands and other countries in Europe, many physicians use decongestants and antihistamines as initial therapy of AOM rather than antibiotics (Chapter 7).

Corticosteroids

Because inflammatory reactions are the main cause of fluid accumulation in the middle ear, a number of studies have evaluated the potential benefits of anti-inflammatory drugs in the management of chronic OME. The oldest and best studied are corticosteroids, administered either orally or by topical nasal spray. Early reports were promising, and recommendations for their use appeared 30 years ago, long before randomized, controlled clinical trials were undertaken. Subsequent investigations have now defined the efficacy and limitations of this therapy.

Generally, topical corticosteroid nasal sprays appear to be effective in a very limited number of children with OME, and although they have not been directly compared to systemic corticosteroid medications, they appear to be less effective. Corticosteroids alone, although shown to be effective in some clinical trials, are more likely to offer benefit when combined with antimicrobial therapy.

The Otitis Media Guideline Panel did not endorse the routine administration of corticosteroids in the management of OME: "Steroid medications are not recommended to treat otitis media with effusion in a child of any age because of limited scientific evidence that this treatment is effective and the opinion of many experts that the possible adverse effects (agitation, behavior change, and more serious problems such as disseminated varicella in children exposed to this virus within the month before therapy) outweighed possible benefits."[6] This conclusion has been questioned because the panel elected to limit its evaluation to the earliest time points in published clinical trials. Early examination in many trials failed to show significant improvement in treatment groups. However, when long-term benefits and cure rates are examined, differences were more significant, and efficacy was better established.

The best evaluation of topical corticosteroid treatment was published by Lildholdt et al,[4] who conducted a double-blind study of beclomethasone nasal spray (Beconase®, Vancenase®) vs placebo in a large group of children with OME. There was no difference in resolution of middle ear fluid for children who received corticosteroids vs the control group. The study was well designed, contained a large number of study patients, and provided optimal follow-up. Although this investigation was undertaken in 1980, additional studies are unlikely to offer more meaningful information.

A meta-analysis of trials evaluating systemic corticosteroids for OME was published by Rosenfeld et al,[14] who critically evaluated 8 large clinical studies. Their conclusion, which contrasts with that of the Otitis Media Guideline Panel, was that systemic corticosteroids were beneficial when combined with antibiotic therapy. They did emphasize that safety data were lacking, and that most studies had some flaws in experimental design.

The most meaningful study and interpretation was offered by Berman,[15] whose clinical trial demonstrated efficacy for a combined antibiotic-corticosteroid regimen. Based on these and other data, the following option for children with OME that persists for 12 weeks or longer seems appropriate: prednisone 0.5-1 mg/kg/d in 1 or 2 divided doses for 7 days, combined with an antibiotic (cephalosporin or macrolide) for 21 days. If this fails—fluid persists for more than 16 weeks and the child has a

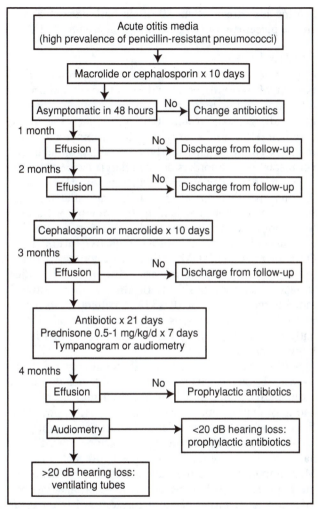

Figure 1: *Algorithm for the management of AOM in geographic regions experiencing a high prevalence of penicillin resistance among clinical isolates of* Streptococcus pneumoniae.

hearing loss greater than 20 dB in both ears—the next step is placement of tympanostomy tubes (Figure 1).

Allergy Control

Researchers believe allergy plays only a minor role in both AOM and OME, because the incidence of otitis media (OM) does not increase in the summer and fall, when inhalant allergens and resultant allergic diatheses are more common. However, allergy may be an important factor for some children, particularly those with prominent upper respiratory symptoms during allergic exacerbations.

All of the evidence linking allergy with OM is indirect: no investigations have clearly demonstrated a convincing pathogenetic mechanism. In addition, conclusions have conflicted in published studies that were designed to examine control of allergy as an adjunctive treatment for OME or recurrent AOM. This lack of consensus likely results from inadequate research design. Many studies showing increased positivity of allergy skin testing or radioallergosorbent test (RAST) in patients with recurrent OM and interventions for these children are inherently biased in that they were usually conducted in allergy referral settings.[16]

Various local respiratory markers for allergy have been shown to be positive in patients with AOM, including nasal eosinophilia, immunoglobulin E (IgE) in middle ear fluid, and mast cells in middle ear mucosa.[17] However, these findings do not confirm cause and effect because they are nonspecific, and other environmental factors may still have had a greater influence in predisposing to acute disease. More importantly, studies have been unable to delineate the sequence of pathologic events to determine whether infection itself might account for some of these local changes before the appearance of allergic manifestations. Perhaps more importantly, clinical trials of allergy control for children with apparent manifestations of allergy and recurrent AOM or OME have failed to clearly dem-

Table 4: Allergy Management to Treat OME: Uncontrolled Clinical Trials and Recommendations

Study	Treatment Intervention	Results
Draper 1974[18]	Hyposensitization intramuscular γ globulin Eustachian tube exercises (yawning, chewing, blowing balloons t.i.d.)	Resolution of middle ear fluid
Kjellman et al 1976[19] (274 children)	Hyposensitization	No benefit
Phillips et al 1974[20]	Antibiotics, nasal decongestants, antihistamines, eustachian tube autoinflation	No benefit
Rapp and Fahey 1973[21]	Topical or oral vasoconstrictors, antihistamines, ventilation techniques (Valsalva's maneuver or politzerization)	50% response

onstrate efficacy, although they have generally reported positive results[18-21] (Table 4). For this reason, the Otitis Media Guideline Panel[6] concluded: "The association between allergy and otitis media with effusion was not clear from available evidence. Thus, although close anatomic relationships between the nasopharynx, eustachian tube, and middle ear have led many experts to suggest a role for allergy management in treating otitis media with effusion, no recommendation was made for or against such treatment."

Myringotomy

Myringotomy was perhaps the first therapy for AOM, introduced by Sir Ashley Cooper in 1802. Thus, until the discovery and availability of antibiotics 130 years later, AOM was considered a surgical rather than a medical disease. Indications for myringotomy are now quite limited. The main consideration centers on its usefulness in managing chronic OME. Otherwise, it is only recommended for the management of acute mastoiditis, labyrinthitis, facial nerve paralysis, and severe otalgia.

Some data, albeit limited, also suggest that myringotomy in conjunction with antimicrobial therapy results in more rapid and consistent resolution of middle ear fluid. However, results have been variable,[22-29] and most studies fail to show benefit. Most convincing was the publication of Qvarnberg et al,[23] who randomized 248 children with AOM into groups treated with antibiotics alone vs antibiotics and myringotomy. In the antibiotic-alone group, 20% more children had persistent middle ear fluid at 2-week follow-up than in the combination group. Ten percent of children who did not undergo myringotomy developed chronic effusions, while this was rare in the myringotomy group. A nonrandomized trial of 158 children with AOM likewise indicated benefit of early myringotomy, particularly in reducing the duration of acute illness.[22] Other published studies failed to demonstrate efficacy (Table 5).

Some studies have shown a higher cure rate for AOM when myringotomy was added to antibiotic therapy.[29] However, the differences are small, and offer real benefit to less than 5% of children. Routine myringotomy for AOM is therefore not indicated.

For many years, myringotomy was a surgical procedure commonly performed by pediatricians and other pri-

Table 5: Myringotomy Plus Antibiotics (MAb) vs Antibiotics Alone (Ab) for Chronic OME

Studies Supporting Myringotomy (*P*<.05)	Persistent Effusion (%)*	
	MAb	Ab
Puhakka et al (1979)[22]	29	78
Qvarnberg et al (1980)[23]	28	50
Studies Not Supporting Myringotomy (*P*>.05)		
Roddey et al (1966)[24]	24	35
Herberts et al (1971)[25]	18	10
Lorentzen et al (1977)[26]	20	16
Schwartz et al (1981)[27]	51	47
Engelhard et al (1989)[28]	40	40
Kaleida et al (1991)[29]	56	61

* Effusion still present 14 days or longer after treatment

mary care physicians to relieve severe otalgia associated with AOM, and less commonly performed to drain persistent middle ear fluid. Published clinical studies have indicated that approximately 1 in 25 children (4%) with AOM have ear pain severe enough to warrant this procedure.[27] Few pediatricians now perform this procedure for a number of good reasons. It should be done by an experienced physician who performs myringotomies more often than a few times each month and who has access to a surgical microscope. Children may need conscious sedation; therefore, facilities must be adequate for management of potential respiratory difficulties. Finally, malpractice insurance rates are considerably higher for physicians who perform this procedure.

Myringotomy has also been carefully evaluated for the management of chronic OME. In two studies conducted at the Otitis Media Research Center at the Children's Hospital of Pittsburgh, Mandel et al[30] stratified and randomly assigned 220 children to treatment with myringotomy plus tube insertion, myringotomy alone, or no surgical intervention. Myringotomy alone offered no advantage over no surgery for the percentage of time with effusion or the number of episodes of AOM. The authors concluded that children with long-standing middle ear effusion should be managed with either watchful waiting and periodic hearing assessment or myringotomy with tube insertion, individualizing the recommendation for each child.

Adenoidectomy and Tonsillectomy

Adenoidectomy, sometimes combined with tonsillectomy, is a surgical approach generally reserved for children who have failed medical management and who have not benefited from tympanostomy tube insertion. The recent increase in the number of adenoidectomies performed in this country, along with the decrease in tonsillectomies, reflect a change in indications and recommendations for these procedures. Rates of adenoidectomy vary considerably by region of the country, likely indicating preferences for management of chronic ear infections.

The first study of tonsillectomy and adenoidectomy and its influence on middle ear disease was reported almost 70 years ago. Since then, a number of other prospective clinical trials have been conducted, with varying results. The larger clinical trials are included in Table 6.[31-35] Benefit is apparently limited to the first year after adenoidectomy, in which the incidence of AOM is reduced. One British study[31] indicated that total AOM episodes were half of that seen in a control group, and a similar study conducted in New Zealand[32] showed a reduction to two thirds of the control incidence.

Table 6: Tonsillectomy/Adenoidectomy (TA) for Recurrent AOM and Chronic OME

Studies Showing Benefit	Outcome Measurement
McKee 1963[31]	Incidence of AOM reduced by 50% in the first year post-TA; no difference the second year.
Roydhouse 1970[32]	Reduction in AOM in the first year post-TA; no difference the second year. Reduced severity of AOM both years.
Maw 1984[33]	One third higher resolution of OME after TA.
Studies Not Showing Benefit	
Kaiser 1930[34]	No difference in the incidence of purulent otorrhea among 4,400 children.
Mawson et al 1967[35]	No difference in the incidence of AOM in 404 children during a 2-year follow-up of TA.

Studies that subsequently examined the relative benefit of tonsillectomy by comparing groups who underwent adenoidectomy plus tonsillectomy versus adenoidectomy alone have failed to show additional benefits of the combined procedure. Most experts have concluded that selective adenoidectomy is the surgical procedure of choice, and that tonsillectomy need only be performed for other indications.

Little information is available concerning tonsillectomy/adenoidectomy for patients with chronic OME. One British study conducted by Maw[33] randomly assigned patients with bilateral chronic OME to undergo adenoidectomy, undergo adenoidectomy and tonsillectomy, or be followed with nonsurgical management. Tympanostomy tubes were placed in one ear with the other ear serving as a control. Only one third of children in the untreated group experienced resolution of their middle ear effusions, while two thirds of patients in both surgical groups became normal during follow-up. Therefore, surgery benefited one third of all children who underwent adenoidectomy or combination procedures.

Tympanostomy Tubes

Only three studies have evaluated the efficacy of tympanostomy tube insertion in preventing recurrences of AOM[36-38] (Table 7). The first, published in 1981 by Gebhart,[36] demonstrated efficacy in prevention of recurrent AOM, but patients were only followed for 6 months. Gonzalez et al[37] followed 65 children with previous recurrent AOM, and concluded that effusions resolve more rapidly after tube placement, but that the overall incidence of AOM recurrences does not decrease. Only infants who had middle ear effusions at the time of enrollment benefited. A larger study of tympanostomy tube placement versus no surgery was conducted by Casselbrant et al,[38] who randomized 264 children between 7 and 35 months old who were otitis media-prone but who did not have OME at the time of entry into the study. The average rate of new episodes per child per year of either AOM or otorrhea was 1.08 in the control group and 1.02 in the tympanostomy tube group ($P=0.25$). However the average proportion of time with OM of any type was 15% in controls and 6.6% in those with tympanostomy tubes ($P<0.001$). The authors concluded that in this young age group, antibiotic chemoprophylaxis was the preferred first measure for preventing recurrences of AOM, and that tympanostomy tubes should be reserved for children who fail medical prophylactic management.

Table 7: Tympanostomy Tubes (TT) for OM

Reason for TT	Results	References
Recurrent AOM	Benefit demonstrated in the prevention of recurrent AOM	Gebhart 1981[36]
	Effusion resolved more rapidly	Gonzalez et al 1986[37]
	No difference in AOM recurrences	
	Reduced % time with AOM; no reduction in total episodes of AOM	Casselbrant et al 1992[38]
Chronic OME	Improved hearing	Marshak et al 1980[39]
	Improvement in hearing and resolution of OME	Gates et al 1987[40]
	Reduced recurrences of AOM	Mandel et al 1989[41]
	More rapid resolution of OME	
	Improved hearing	

Several studies have examined the efficacy of tympanostomy tube placement for the treatment for chronic OME. Three recent ones are included in Table 7.[39-41] All showed improved hearing after the surgical procedure, and the two studies that monitored resolution of middle ear fluid showed more rapid responses after this surgical procedure. The study by Mandel et al[41] was designed for long-term follow-up of 109 children who had been unresponsive to prophylactic antimicrobial therapy. Patients were followed for 3 years with monthly evaluations. AOM recurrence was significantly reduced. Many of the other children in this study who had undergone only myringotomies, or who were followed in a control group, required tympanostomy tube insertion because of progressive hearing loss. Half of the children with tympanostomy tubes had episodes of otorrhea during the course of follow-up, but these usually resolved with short-course antimicrobial therapy. One child in the surgical treatment group required bilateral tympanoplasties to treat chronic tympanic membrane perforations that persisted after the tubes were extruded. A second phase of this study[30] included 111 children randomized to myringotomy, myringotomy and tympanostomy tube insertion, and a no-surgery control group. Similar to the first study, all patients were carefully followed monthly for 3 years. This follow-up study confirmed results from the first series, in that subjects who underwent myringotomy and tube replacement had less time with middle ear effusion and better hearing than the myringotomy or control cases. The authors concluded that children with chronic OME unresponsive to medical therapy that persists for 4 months or longer undergo myringotomy and tympanostomy tube placement. They further advised reserving adenoidectomy for patients who did not benefit from tympanostomy tubes.

References

1. Collipp PJ: Evaluation of nose drops for otitis media in children. *Northwest Med* 1961;60:999-1000.

2. Fraser JG, Mehta M, Fraser PA: The medical treatment of secretory otitis media. A clinical trial of three commonly used regimes. *J Laryngol Otol* 1977;91:757-765.

3.   Cantekin EI, Bluestone CD, Rockette HE, et al: Effect of oral decongestant with or without antihistamine on eustachian tube function. *Ann Otol Rhinol Laryngol Suppl* 1980;89:290-295.

4.   Lildholdt T, Cantekin EI, Bluestone CD, et al: Effect of topical nasal decongestant on eustachian tube function in children with tympanostomy tubes. *Acta Otolaryngol (Stockh)* 1982;94:93-97.

5.   Schwartz RH, Schwartz DM: Acute otitis media: diagnosis and drug therapy. *Drugs* 1980;19:107-118.

6.   The Otitis Media Guideline Panel of the American Academy of Pediatrics: Managing otitis media with effusion in young children. *Pediatrics* 1994;94:766-773.

7.   Rubenstein MM, McBean JB, Hedgecock LD, et al: The treatment of acute otitis media in children. III. A third clinical trial. *Am J Dis Child* 1965;109:308-313.

8.   Miller GF: Influence of an oral decongestant on eustachian tube function in children. *J Allergy* 1970;45:187-193.

9.   Stickler GB, Rubenstein MM, McBean JB, et al: Treatment of acute otitis media in children. IV. A fourth clinical trial. *Am J Dis Child* 1967;114:123-130.

10. Olson AL, Klein SW, Charney E, et al: Prevention and therapy of serous otitis media by oral decongestant: a double-blind study in pediatric practice. *Pediatrics* 1978;61:679-684.

11. Holmquist J: Medical treatment in ears with eustachian tube dysfunction. Presented at the Symposium on Physiology and Pathophysiology of the Eustachian Tube and Middle Ear, September 28, 1977, Freiburg, West Germany.

12. Cantekin EI, Mandel EM, Bluestone CD, et al: Lack of efficacy of a decongestant-antihistamine combination for otitis media with effusion ("secretory" otitis media) in children. Results of a double-blind, randomized trial. *N Engl J Med* 1983;308:297-301.

13. Mandel EM, Rockette HE, Bluestone CD, et al: Efficacy of amoxicillin with and without decongestant-antihistamine for otitis media with effusion in children. Results of a double-blind, randomized trial. *N Engl J Med* 1987;316:432-437.

14. Rosenfeld RM, Mandel EM, Bluestone CD: Systemic steroids for otitis media with effusion in children. *Arch Otolaryngol Head Neck Surg* 1991;117:984-989.

15. Berman S: Medical management of children with otitis media with effusion. *Rep Pediatr Infect Dis* 1993;3:37-38.

16. Mogi G: Immunologic and allergic aspects of otitis media. In: Lim DJ, Bluestone CD, Klein JO, et al, eds. *Recent Advances in Otitis Media with Effusion.* Burlington, Ontario, Decker Periodicals, 1993, pp 145-151.

17. Bernstein JM: The role of IgE-mediated hypersensitivity in the development of otitis media with effusion. *Otolaryngol Clin North Am* 1992;25:197-211.

18. Draper WL: Allergy in relationship to the eustachian tube and middle ear. *Otolaryngol Clin North Am* 1974;7:749-755.

19. Kjellman NI, Synnerstad B, Hansson LO: Atopic allergy and immunoglobulins in children with adenoids and recurrent otitis media. *Acta Paediatr Scand* 1976;65:593-600.

20. Phillips MJ, Knight NJ, Manning H, et al: IgE and secretory otitis media. *Lancet* 1974;2:1176-1178.

21. Rapp DJ, Fahey D: Review of chronic secretory otitis and allergy. *J Asthma Res* 1973;10:193-218.

22. Puhakka H, Virolainen E, Aantaa E, et al: Myringotomy in the treatment of acute otitis media in children. *Acta Otolaryngol (Stockh)* 1979;88:122-126.

23. Qvarnberg Y, Palva T: Active and conservative treatment of acute otitis media. Prospective studies. *Ann Otol Rhinol Laryngol Suppl* 1980;89:269-270.

24. Roddey OF Jr, Earle R Jr, Haggerty R: Myringotomy in acute otitis media. A controlled study. *JAMA* 1966;197:849-853.

25. Herberts G, Jeppsson PH, Nylen O, et al: Acute otitis media. Etiologic and therapeutic aspects of acute otitis media. *Pract Otorhinolaryngol (Basel)* 1971;33:191-202.

26. Lorentzen P, Haugsten P: Treatment of acute suppurative otitis media. *J Laryngol Otol* 1977;91:331-340.

27. Schwartz RH, Rodriguez WG, Schwartz DM: Office myringotomy for acute otitis media: its value in preventing middle ear effusion. *Laryngoscope* 1981;91:616-619.

28. Engelhard D, Cohen D, Strauss N, et al: Randomised study of myringotomy, amoxycillin/clavulanate, or both for acute otitis media in infants. *Lancet* 1989;2:141-143.

29. Kaleida PH, Casselbrant ML, Rockette HE, et al: Amoxicillin or myringotomy or both for acute otitis media: results of a randomized clinical trial. *Pediatrics* 1991;87:466-474.

30. Mandel EM, Rockette HE, Bluestone CD, et al: Efficacy of myringotomy with and without tympanostomy tubes for chronic otitis media with effusion. *Pediatr Infect Dis J* 1992;11:270-277.

31. McKee WJ: A controlled study of the effects of tonsillectomy and adenoidectomy in children. *Br J Prev Soc Med* 1963;17:46-49.

32. Roydhouse N: A controlled study of adenotonsillectomy. *Arch Otolaryngol* 1970;92:611-616.

33. Maw AR: Chronic otitis media with effusion and adenotonsillectomy: a prospective randomized controlled study. In: Lim DJ, Bluestone CD, Klein JO, et al, eds. *Recent Advances in Otitis Media with Effusion.* Toronto, BC Decker, 1984, pp 299-302.

34. Kaiser AD: Results of tonsillectomy: a comparative study of 2,200 tonsillectomized children with an equal number of controls three and ten years after operation. *JAMA* 1930;95:837-842.

35. Mawson SR, Adlington R, Evans M: A controlled study evaluation of adeno-tonsillectomy in children. *J Laryngol Otol* 1967;81:777-790.

36. Gebhart DE: Tympanostomy tubes in the otitis media prone child. *Laryngoscope* 1981;91:849-866.

37. Gonzalez C, Arnold JE, Woody EA, et al: Prevention of recurrent acute otitis media: chemoprophylaxis versus tympanostomy tubes. *Laryngoscope* 1986;96:1330-1334.

38. Casselbrant ML, Kaleida PH, Rockette HE, et al: Efficacy of antimicrobial prophylaxis and of tympanostomy tube insertion for prevention of recurrent acute otitis media: results of a randomized clinical trial. *Pediatr Infect Dis J* 1992;11:278-286.

39. Marshak G, Neriah ZB: Adenoidectomy versus tympanostomy in chronic secretory otitis media. *Ann Otol Rhinol Laryngol Suppl* 1980;89:316-318.

40. Gates GA, Avery CA, Prihoda TJ, et al: Effectiveness of adenoidectomy and tympanostomy tubes in the treatment of chronic otitis media with effusion. *N Engl J Med* 1987;317:1444-1451.

41. Mandel EM, Rockette HE, Bluestone CD, et al: Myringotomy with and without tympanostomy tubes for chronic otitis media with effusion. *Arch Otolaryngol Head Neck Surg* 1989;115:1217-1224.

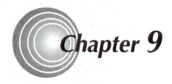

Chapter 9

The Otitis Media-Prone Child

Clinical histories of young children indicate three patterns relative to their childhood experiences with otitis media, and that approximately one third of all children fall into each of these categories.[1,2] The first group includes children who remain free from any episodes of acute otitis media (AOM) in the first 3 years of life. These children are more likely to be cared for at home rather than at day-care centers. Family histories are generally negative for cigarette smoking and indicate a low incidence of ear infections in siblings and parents. Another third of all children have 1 or 2 episodes of AOM in the first 3 years of life, which readily respond to antimicrobial therapy followed by rapid resolution of middle ear effusions. The third group is usually referred to as otitis media-prone children, a term originally suggested by Howie et al.[1] These individuals have 3 or more episodes of AOM in early childhood, with the first episode often occurring before 6 months of age. They commonly have siblings with repeated middle ear infection and are more likely to be cared for in large day-care centers. Middle ear effusions are often slow to resolve in these children, and they need special management for chronic middle ear changes. Other epidemiologic factors that might predispose children to the otitis media-prone condition are addressed in Chapter 1 and summarized in Table 1, along with universal intervention strategies recommended for all children beginning at birth.

Table 1: Risk Factors for Recurrent Acute Otitis Media (AOM)

Factors we can influence

- Bottle propping
- Parental smoking
- Total bottle feeding
- Anatomic defects (cleft palate)
- Immune deficiency
- Inadequate medical care
- Poor sanitation

Factors we may influence

- Large-group day care
- Poverty
- Crowded living conditions

Factors we cannot influence

- Male gender
- Ethnic groups (American Indian, Eskimos)
- First episode at early age
- First episode caused by *Streptococcus pneumoniae*
- Sibling or parental history of recurrent AOM
- Season (winter, fall)

Definition

Published clinical studies related to recurrent AOM have defined the otitis-prone condition in a number of different ways.[1-5] These definitions were generally used to identify children expected to have frequent episodes of middle ear disease, and for whom study interventions were

Table 2: Definitions of the Otitis Media-Prone Child

- 3 episodes of AOM in 6 months
- 4 episodes of AOM in 12 months
- 1 episode before 6 months old

    plus

    an otitis media-prone sibling
- 2 episodes in the first year of life

being examined. Recurrent AOM is assumed to be associated with persistent otitis media with effusion (OME), which ultimately results in significant interference with cognitive development.

Table 2 outlines definitions for the otitis media-prone child based on the total number of episodes over defined periods of time, and on some additional factors that help predict which children might have recurrent AOM. Surveys of practicing pediatricians indicate that most define the otitis media-prone child as one who has had 3 episodes of otitis media (OM) in a 6-month period. With this definition, approximately 40% of all children in an average office practice would be managed with the interventions recommended for such patients. The most strict definition used by some physicians is 6 episodes of OM in the first year of life. Clinical surveys indicate that approximately 1 in 7 children experience AOM this frequently. Although a single episode of AOM before 6 months of age carries a high risk for subsequent recurrent infection, frequent infections really only follow when this episode is caused by *Streptococcus pneumoniae*. Unless a tympanocentesis is performed to identify the responsible pathogen, information for a specific etiol-

ogy is not available. Therefore, this definition is not prac-
tical in the usual office setting.

Groups of children for whom preventive interventions, particularly antibiotic chemoprophylaxis, are recommended even before a first episode of OM include cleft palate, Navajo Indians, Apache Indians, Eskimos, Down syndrome, and Turner's syndrome. Perhaps the largest group encountered in general practice are children whose siblings were otitis media-prone. Once the younger child has an episode of AOM before 6 months of age, many experts recommend immediate interventions to prevent recurrent disease.

Management

Most primary care physicians use a sequential approach to management of the otitis media-prone child, as outlined in Table 3. Many experts recommend proceeding stepwise until recurrent episodes of AOM are controlled and middle ear effusion has resolved. A simple yet extremely important initial management step for the otitis media-prone child is control of environmental risk factors. Adequate scientific data show that the following factors potentially increase the risks for recurrent AOM or OME: bottle-feeding rather than breast-feeding infants; passive smoking; and group child-care attendance. The first risk factor, breast-feeding, cannot usually be altered, since otitis media-prone children are generally not identified until late infancy or early childhood, long after decisions for method of feeding have been made.

Passive smoking (exposure to another's tobacco smoke) is associated with a higher risk of OME. Although there is no proof that eliminating passive smoking helps prevent recurrent AOM or OME, there are many health reasons for not exposing persons of any age to tobacco smoke. Therefore, clinicians should advise parents of the benefits of decreasing children's exposure to tobacco smoke.

Table 3: Sequential Management of the Otitis Media-Prone Child

- Environmental control
- Antibiotic prophylaxis
- Pneumococcal and influenza vaccines
- Combination therapy (Chapter 10)
- Tympanostomy tubes
- Adenoidectomy

Studies of OME in children cared for at home compared to those in group child-care facilities found that children in group child-care facilities have a slightly higher relative risk (less than 2.0) of OME. Studies have not been undertaken, however, to examine whether removing children from group child-care facilities prevents OME.

The mainstay for managing the otitis media-prone child and preventing subsequent episodes of AOM is antibiotic prophylaxis. Many well-designed clinical trials have supported their use, and these subsequently resulted in drug labeling indications approved by the Food and Drug Administration (FDA).[6] Candidates for this preventive intervention should fulfill criteria for being otitis media-prone as defined in Table 2, and must also fulfill the following additional requirements: age less than 2 years, no current effusion, no gastrointestinal absorption limitations, and assurance of compliance. Studies that have demonstrated significant benefit from antibiotic prophylaxis are described in detail in Chapter 10.

Antimicrobial agents that have been used for chemoprophylaxis are included in Table 4. Most studies have used a sulfonamide, most prominently sulfisoxazole, but studies with trimethoprim/sulfamethoxazole (TMP/SMX, Bactrim™, Septra®), amoxicillin, and erythromycin have also supported these agents for prophylactic use in otitis media-prone children.[7] TMP/SMX is not recommended for infants younger than 2 months and, although this antibiotic combination is approved for the treatment of AOM in children, it is not indicated for prophylactic or prolonged administration for OM at any age, despite clinical studies that have supported its efficacy. This is because the FDA was not convinced that efficacy data for prophylaxis were adequate.

Amoxicillin is much less popular for prophylaxis because of the markedly increased resistance of pneumococci to penicillin antibiotics.[8] If amoxicillin is selected, a higher dosage should be used, as indicated in Table 5. In the past, the prophylactic dose of amoxicillin was generally 15 to 20 mg/kg, but this dosage is now unlikely to be effective for more than 50% of pneumococci. A dosage of 30 to 45 mg/kg should be effective against 70% to 80% of pneumococci whose minimum inhibitory concentration (MIC) is below 2 µg/mL. On the other hand, results from the 1997 antimicrobial surveillance program in North America indicate that 89% of *Streptococcus pneumoniae* are susceptible to TMP/SMX, and that more than 80% are susceptible to other sulfonamides.[9] These recent data well support the continued use of sulfisoxazole as chemoprophylaxis for children with recurrent AOM.

Most studies indicate that maximum benefit is provided to infants and children younger than 2 years old as long as compliance is achieved. Also, most studies have a carryover effect in that once children are off any particular prophylactic regimen, they are still relatively disease-free for a few months after terminating the antibiotic.

Recent studies indicate that drug resistance emerges fairly rapidly during the course of antimicrobial chemoprophylaxis, as judged by the susceptibility patterns of pathogens that potentially colonize the posterior nasopharynx during chemoprophylaxis or for a few months after-

Table 4: Preventive Interventions for the Otitis Media-Prone Child

Chemoprophylaxis

- sulfisoxazole
- sulfamethoxazole
- TMP/SMX
- erythromycin/sulfisoxazole
- amoxicillin
- ampicillin
- penicillin

Pneumococcal and influenza vaccines

Xylitol sugar

- chewing gum
- lozenge
- syrup

Middle ear inflation

Surgical procedures

- tympanostomy tubes
- adenoidectomy

ward.[8] These data are troublesome, and warrant careful continued attention.

Because one objective in managing the otitis media-prone child is elimination of middle ear effusions, patients on chemoprophylaxis should be examined periodically. If effusion persists, additional interventions may be warranted, and are outlined in Chapter 11. The clinician should consider offering a short course of corticosteroid therapy along with therapeutic doses of antibiotics just before beginning a longer regimen of chemoprophylaxis. Routine use of corticosteroids remains somewhat controversial and should probably be individualized, taking into account the patient's age, degree of hearing loss, and duration of OME, before beginning other interventions.

Research protocols have used different timing and duration of antibiotic chemoprophylaxis. These include continuous use of antibiotics for 90 days after the episode of AOM that defined the child as otitis media-prone, continuous use of chemoprophylaxis during the winter months (usually November through March), or intermittent prophylaxis when the child has a viral upper respiratory infection. With the latter approach, therapy is continued for 5 to 8 days, the usual duration of respiratory infections. No method can be interpreted as significantly better than others because few comparative trials of this variable have been conducted. However, the studies that have compared different methods of timing and duration for chemoprophylaxis generally conclude that continuous daily therapy is superior to intermittent prophylaxis.[10] No differences are apparent between a continuous protocol that is begun after the child is determined to be otitis media-prone, and one that is designed to administer chemoprophylaxis during the winter months. Agreement is growing among practicing clinicians to offer preventive therapy for 3 months after a child has fulfilled an acceptable definition for otitis-prone. This usually means that antibiotics will be continued at prophylactic dosages after the child completes a course of therapy for an acute episode. These children should then be seen every 6 to 8 weeks until middle ear fluid is resolved or until they have completed their trial of prophylactic antibiotics.

Other Preventive Interventions

A few other medical procedures and a number of surgical approaches have been examined for management of the otitis media-prone child, and these are listed in Table

4 and reviewed in more detail in Chapter 10. Pneumococ-cal[11,12] and influenza[13] vaccines warrant consideration not only for the otitis media-prone child, but also as a universal preventive intervention. Xylitol sugar used as a chewing gum, syrup, or lozenge appears to be effective,[14] but is impractical, and products that contain adequate amounts of xylitol for this purpose are not available in the United States. Middle ear inflation is certainly an inexpensive procedure that might offer benefit to a small number of children, but has not appeared effective in controlled clinical trials.[15]

Tympanostomy tubes are now the most popular surgical procedure usually offered to children who fail antibiotic chemoprophylaxis.[16,17] This surgical step is generally recommended for patients who have persistent middle ear effusion lasting longer than 4 to 6 months and who have a hearing loss greater than 20 dB in both ears. Data supporting efficacy of tympanostomy tubes are provided in Chapter 10, and a review of the surgical aspects of tympanostomy tube placement appears in Chapter 13.

Adenoidectomy is a surgical intervention that has been recommended for children with recurrent AOM, but is generally reserved for patients who fail medical management and who do not improve after tympanostomy tube insertion. Benefit appears limited to the first year after adenoidectomy, when the total incidence of AOM is reduced. This incidence may be as low as one third to one half of those episodes experienced by children who do not undergo this procedure. Published clinical trials demonstrating efficacy are reviewed in Chapter 10, and surgical issues related to adenoidectomy are outlined in Chapter 13. Tonsillectomy has also been examined as a potential surgical step for these children, but has never been shown to influence the overall incidence of recurrent AOM. Tonsillectomy should only be recommended in conjunction with adenoidectomy if there are other indications for removing the tonsils.

References

1. Howie VM, Ploussard JH, Sloyer J: The "otitis-prone" condition. *Am J Dis Child* 1975;129:676-678.

2. Teele DW, Klein JO, Rosner B: Epidemiology of otitis media during the first seven years of life in children in greater Boston: a prospective, cohort study. *J Infect Dis* 1989;160:83-94.

3. Alho OP, Koivu M, Sorri M, et al: Risk factors for recurrent acute otitis media and respiratory infection in infancy. *Int J Pediatr Otorhinolaryngol* 1990;19:151-161.

4. Alho OP, Koivu M, Sorri M: What is an 'otitis-prone' child? *Int J Pediatr Otorhinolaryngol* 1991;21:201-209.

5. Klein JO: Otitis media. *Clin Infect Dis* 1994;19:823-833.

6. Liston TE, Foshee WS, Pierson WD: Sulfisoxazole chemoprophylaxis for frequent otitis media. *Pediatrics* 1983;71:524-530.

7. Principi N, Marchisio P, Massironi E, et al: Prophylaxis of recurrent acute otitis media and middle-ear effusion. Comparison of amoxicillin with sulfamethoxazole and trimethoprim. *Am J Dis Child* 1989;143:1414-1418.

8. Dowell SF, Marcy SM, Phillips WR, et al: Otitis media—principles of judicious use of antimicrobial agents. *Pediatrics* 1998;101:S165-S171.

9. Doern GV, Pfaller MA, Kugler K, et al: Prevalence of antimicrobial resistance among respiratory tract isolates of *Streptococcus pneumoniae* in North America: 1997 results from the SENTRY antimicrobial surveillance program. *Clin Infect Dis* 1998;27:764-770.

10. Berman S, Nuss R, Roark R, et al: Effectiveness of continuous vs. intermittent amoxicillin to prevent episodes of otitis media. *Pediatr Infect Dis J* 1992;11:63-67.

11. Rennels MB, Edwards KM, Keyserling HC, et al: Safety and immunogenicity of heptavalent pneumococcal vaccine conjugated to CRM_{197} in United States infants. *Pediatrics* 1998;101:604-611.

12. Sloyer JL Jr, Ploussard JH, Howie VM: Efficacy of pneumococcal polysaccharide vaccine in preventing acute otitis media in infants in Huntsville, Alabama. *Rev Infect Dis* 1981;3:S119-S123.

13. Heikkinen T, Ruuskanen O, Waris M, et al: Influenza vaccination in the prevention of acute otitis media in children. *Am J Dis Child* 1991;145:445-448.

14. Uhari M, Kontiokari T, Niemela M: A novel use of xylitol sugar in preventing acute otitis media. *Pediatrics* 1998;102: 879-884.

15. Chan KH, Bluestone CD: Lack of efficacy of middle-ear inflation: treatment of otitis media with effusion in children. *Otolaryngol Head Neck Surg* 1989;100:317-323.

16. Casselbrant ML, Kaleida PH, Rockette HE, et al: Efficacy of antimicrobial prophylaxis and of tympanostomy tube insertion for prevention of recurrent acute otitis media: results of a randomized clinical trial. *Pediatr Infect Dis J* 1992;11:278-286.

17. Gonzalez C, Arnold JE, Woody EA, et al: Prevention of recurrent acute otitis media: chemoprophylaxis versus tympanostomy tubes. *Laryngoscope* 1986;96:1330-1334.

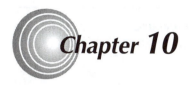

Chapter 10

Prevention

B ecause otitis media (OM) is so common (Chapter 1), every effort must be made to routinely implement preventive measures as early as possible during childhood. Some of these measures, such as elimination of bottle propping and environmental control (Table 1), are relatively simple. Administration of vaccines that might prevent disease caused by specific middle ear pathogens, such as *Streptococcus pneumoniae*, is an additional strategy that may be considered, although data supporting efficacy are not yet complete.[1] The conjugate *Haemophilus influenzae* type b vaccine, on the other hand, has essentially eliminated invasive *H influenzae* disease, including OM, but only 10% of all *H influenzae* OM is caused by type b pathogens. The remainder, approximately 90%, is attributable to nontypeable strains that are not affected by *H influenzae* vaccine. Therefore, this vaccine has had very little impact on the overall incidence of acute otitis media (AOM). If the conjugate pneumococcal vaccines are as effective as conjugate *H influenzae* products, the epidemiology of middle ear disease is likely to change considerably.

Influenza viruses are highly associated with AOM, and prevention of these viral diseases with vaccine has been shown to reduce the incidence of bacterial AOM during influenza outbreaks.[2] Similarly, AOM associated with respiratory syncytial virus (RSV) infection can be reduced with the prophylactic administration of either intravenous RSV hyperimmune globulin (RespiGam®) or intramus-

Table 1: Routine Measures to Prevent Recurrent AOM

- Breast-feeding
- Eliminate bottle propping
- Environmental control
  — Avoid smoking inside the home
  — Limit large day-care attendance
- Pneumococcal conjugate vaccine
- Influenza vaccine
- *Haemophilus influenzae* type b vaccine

cular RSV monoclonal antibody (palivizumab, Synagis™).[3] Candidates for these extremely expensive preventive measures are children born at gestational ages <32 weeks or those with bronchopulmonary dysplasia. Therapy for such high-risk children is not specifically directed at the prevention of AOM, but rather at the control of RSV pulmonary disease, which can be life-threatening in these populations.

The most important epidemiologic factor is day-care center attendance, particularly large-group facilities. The risk results from the constant and close exposure to other young children who may harbor respiratory pathogens and transmit them to their susceptible playmates. Epidemics of viral disease are quite common in this setting, transmitted not only by coughing or sneezing, but also by contamination of fomites. Observations of toddlers in day-care environments have shown that these children place some object in their mouths more frequently than once every minute. At this age, children are quite sharing with other children and, of course, are too young to understand the risks of such behavior.

Table 2: The Otitis Media-Prone Child: Definitions and Requirements for Chemoprophylaxis

Definition

- 3 episodes of AOM within 6 months
- 4 episodes of AOM within 12 months
- 1 episode before 6 months of age

    plus

    an otitis media-prone sibling

- 2 episodes in the first year of life

Requirements

- Under 2 years old
- No current effusion (see Chapter 11)
- No gastrointestinal absorption limitations
- Compliance assured

Respiratory pathogens such as RSV and rhinovirus may remain viable for hours or even days on fomites such as toys, particularly if they remain moist from secretions. The sharing of these toys by children greatly increases the potential for colonization with viral pathogens. For this reason, washing and drying of toys at least daily is recommended as routine policy in child-care facilities.

The Otitis Media-Prone Child

Approximately one third of all children have repeated episodes of acute middle ear infection. This clinical problem is identified in the medical literature as 'the otitis media-prone child.' Management of children with recurrent AOM is addressed in detail in Chapter 9, and the accepted definitions of the otitis media-prone child are sum-

Table 3: Preventive Interventions for the Otitis Media-Prone Child

Chemoprophylaxis

- sulfisoxazole
- sulfamethoxazole
- trimethoprim/sulfamethoxazole (TMP/SMX)
- sulfisoxazole/erythromycin
- amoxicillin
- ampicillin
- penicillin

Xylitol sugar

- chewing gum
- lozenge
- syrup

Middle ear inflation

Surgical procedures

- tympanostomy tubes
- adenoidectomy

marized in Table 2. Such classification for these children is important primarily because specific management steps have been examined and have been shown to provide benefit in preventing recurrent episodes of AOM, and in preventing progression of chronic middle ear disease (Table 3). Most importantly, these children are appropriate candidates for antibiotic chemoprophylaxis once they fulfill additional requirements (Table 2).

Older studies in the 1970s and 1980s indicated that, in the outpatient setting, 1 in 7 children are expected to have

> ## Table 4: Options for Antibiotic Chemoprophylaxis
>
> - 90 days after the last episode of AOM
> - During the winter months (November to March)
> - During any apparent viral upper respiratory infection (URI) (5 to 8 days)

more than 6 episodes of OM during the first 2 years of life.[4] Other studies have indicated that almost half of all children have 3 or more episodes by 3 years of age.[5] Age at the time of the first episode of AOM is highly correlated with recurrences: two thirds of children with a first episode before 6 months old will have 3 or more episodes in the following 6 months. In contrast, a child whose first episode is diagnosed after 1 year of age has only a 26% probability of being otitis media-prone. Additional categories of children who are highly predisposed to recurrent AOM are addressed in Chapter 1. These include certain ethnic groups (eg, American Indians, Eskimos), and children with genetic abnormalities such as Down syndrome and Turner's syndrome. Recurrent disease is so common in these children that many experts recommend chemoprophylaxis even before they have had their first episode of AOM.

Antibiotic Chemoprophylaxis

For many years, the primary medical approach to the management of recurrent AOM has been antibiotic chemoprophylaxis. Many well-designed clinical trials have supported their use, and subsequently resulted in drug labeling indications approved by the Food and Drug Administration (FDA). Candidates for this preventive intervention should meet strict criteria that define the otitis media-prone child, and should also fulfill other requirements (Table 2). One concern is that the daily low dos-

Table 5: Sulfonamide Chemoprophylaxis for the Prevention of Recurrent Otitis Media

Antibiotic	Timing and Duration of Chemoprophylaxis; Study Design	Reference
Sulfisoxazole	December to May Placebo-controlled b.i.d. dosing	Perrin et al (1974)[6]
	During viral URI b.i.d. dosing	Biedel (1978)[7]
	3 months Double-blind crossover b.i.d. dosing	Liston, et al (1983)[8]
	Continual 1 to 2 years b.i.d. dosing	Schuller (1983)[9]
	Winter months Double-blind crossover b.i.d. dosing	Varsano et al (1985)[10]
	6 months b.i.d. dosing	Gonzalez et al (1986)[11]

ages of antibiotics normally recommended for prophylaxis might increase the antimicrobial resistance of common middle ear pathogens, particularly if amoxicillin is used. Therefore, benefits for a particular patient must be carefully weighed against the consequence of increasing bacterial resistance. In light of this problem, recent guideline

Antibiotic	Timing and Duration of Chemoprophylaxis; Study Design	Reference
Sulfamethoxazole	2 months total Double-blind crossover Once-daily dosing	Schwartz et al (1982)[12]
Sulfisoxazole vs erythromycin	2 months total b.i.d. dosing (benefit only seen with erythromycin)	Lampe et al (1986)[13]
Trimethoprim/ sulfamethoxazole (TMP/SMX)	3 months total Once-daily dosing	Gray (1981)[14]

recommendations have suggested that chemoprophylaxis be reserved for children under 2 years old,[15] since younger patients are more likely to benefit, and that antimicrobial therapy not be used for otitis media with effusion (OME).

Research protocols have varied regarding timing and duration of antibiotic chemoprophylaxis (Table 4). No method can be interpreted as significantly better than another, since few comparative trials of this variable have been conducted. However, those studies that compared different methods of timing and duration for chemoprophylaxis generally conclude that continuous daily therapy is superior to intermittent prophylaxis. There appears to be no difference between a continuous protocol that is begun after the child is determined to be otitis media-prone, and one that is designed to administer chemoprophylaxis during the winter months. A popular option is to offer preventive therapy for 3 months after a child has fulfilled definitions for being otitis media-prone. This usually means that antibiotics will be continued at prophylactic dosages after the child completes a course of therapy for an acute episode. These children should then be seen every 6 to 8 weeks until middle ear fluid is resolved or until they have completed their trial of antibiotics.

Tables 5 and 6 summarize published clinical trials that have examined the usefulness of antimicrobial chemoprophylaxis for children with recurrent AOM. Most of these studies employed sulfisoxazole or another sulfonamide, and these particular publications are included in Table 5. Virtually all clinical studies have demonstrated at least some degree of therapeutic efficacy in patients receiving chemoprophylaxis. Patients who particularly benefited were those children who had frequent episodes of AOM and who were under 2 years old when antibiotic prophylaxis was begun. These children generally experienced a reduction in total episodes of AOM to approximately one third of that documented in control patients, or in episodes that occurred during the control periods in the studies that were double blind and crossover. Approximately one half of children on chemoprophylaxis were also observed to be totally free from subsequent episodes of OM, and attained normal or at least satisfactory eustachian tube function. Interestingly, benefit usually persisted for at least several months after

Table 6: Other Antibiotic Chemoprophylaxis for the Prevention of Recurrent Otitis Media

Antibiotic	Timing and Duration of Chemoprophylaxis	Reference
Amoxicillin	6 months Once-daily dosing	Principi et al (1989)[16]
	Continuous or during the winter months (depending on history) Once-daily dosing	Casselbrant et al (1992)[17]
	During the winter months (4 months total) or with viral URI b.i.d. dosing	Berman et al (1992)[18]
Ampicillin	1 year Once-daily dosing	Maynard et al (1972)[19]
Penicillin	Continuous Once-daily dosing	Persico et al (1978)[20]

cessation of prophylaxis. As expected, a small percentage of children on antibiotics developed some adverse reactions to medication, but these were rarely serious. One consistent finding, and the one of greatest concern, is the change in antibiotic susceptibility of colonizing organisms, such as pneumococci, and their increased resistance to the class of antibiotics used for prophylaxis.

The dosages of antibiotics for prophylaxis are generally one half of those used for therapy: sulfisoxazole 50 to 75 mg/kg; sulfamethoxazole 25 mg/kg; trimethoprim/

sulfamethoxazole (TMP/SMX, Bactrim™, Septra®) 10 to 12 mg/kg, and amoxicillin 30 to 45 mg/kg. They can be given once a day or divided b.i.d.; both approaches have been used in clinical trials. Acute infections that occur during the course of chemoprophylaxis should be treated similarly to an episode in patients not on preventive therapy. Prophylaxis should then be continued after completing therapy for the intercurrent infection. Pathogens in this circumstance are, of course, highly likely to be resistant to the antibiotic used for prophylaxis.

Xylitol Sugar

Xylitol is a 5-carbon polyol that is used extensively in Europe as a sweetening substitute for sucrose because it has been shown to prevent dental caries. This beneficial effect results from an inhibition of growth of *Streptococcus mutans*, the bacterium that is primarily responsible for tooth decay. Xylitol has also been shown to inhibit the growth of *S pneumoniae*, and for this reason was examined for its ability to prevent OM.

In a study conducted in Finland, 857 healthy children in day-care centers were enrolled in a trial designed to examine the potential benefits of xylitol syrup, xylitol gum, and xylitol lozenges.[21] The study was conducted for 3 months, during which time study patients received xylitol 5 times daily. Xylitol syrup reduced the incidence of AOM by 30% and chewing gum by 40%. The overall need for antimicrobial therapy was also significantly reduced. Although xylitol lozenges decreased episodes of AOM by 20%, this was not statistically significant. Thus, xylitol as either a chewable gum in older children or a syrup in younger children significantly lowered the occurrence of AOM and the requirement for antimicrobials; the latter benefit pertained to the use of antibiotics for ear infections as well as other indications.

Chewing gum in the United States contains relatively low amounts of xylitol but relatively large amounts of sorbitol. Because gastrointestinal side effects are common after ingestion of large amounts of sorbitol, it is unlikely that available products could be used to deliver xylitol. The other main shortcoming of this approach is compliance. Two pieces of gum must be chewed for at least 5 minutes, 5 times a day. Young children are unlikely to tolerate this. Likewise, giving oral medications 5 times a day is impractical.

Middle Ear Inflation

Procedures that provide mechanisms for opening the middle-ear cavity and eustachian tubes have been used for decades as adjunctive measures for eliminating effusion. Most popular are Valsalva's maneuver and another described by Politzer in 1909, subsequently termed politzerization. However, clinical trials have indicated that these procedures are unlikely to offer significant benefit for eliminating middle-ear fluid in a large number of children.[22] Some experts argue that self-inflation is a simple procedure without any additional cost, and therefore could be instituted for a limited time in more difficult cases that have failed standard therapeutic approaches.

Valsalva's maneuver requires forced nasal expiration while the nose is pinched and the mouth is also closed. This maneuver is difficult for children less than 6 years old. The method described by Politzer requires participation by parents. A rubber air bulb is introduced into one nostril while the other nostril is closed off by digital pressure. The child then swallows while the rubber bulb is compressed. This produces a sudden opening of the middle ear when air is rapidly introduced, and therefore may be somewhat uncomfortable. Success of these procedures can be partly documented if the child is old enough to describe the ears 'popping.' After success with the Valsalva maneuver or politzerization, bubbles or an air-fluid level may be seen as a new finding on physical examination. Evidence of improvement on a tympanogram, with a shift

Table 7: Pneumococcal Polysaccharide Vaccine for the Prevention of Recurrent AOM

Reference	Results
Karma et al (1980)[23]	Protection against vaccine strains in infants >6 months
Makela et al (1981)[24]	Overall reduction of AOM 2 to 5 years of age
Sloyer et al (1981)[25]	Lower incidence of AOM after 1 year of age
Teele et al (1981)[26]	No difference in overall AOM Reduction in vaccine types of pneumococcus
Rosen et al (1983)[27]	Reduced clinical AOM
Howie et al (1984)[28]	Reduction of AOM in black children 6 to 11 months of age No benefits in white infants

of the compliance peak toward the positive pressure zone, would be more important.

Pneumococcal Polysaccharide Vaccine

Some data, albeit limited, suggest that pneumococcal polysaccharide vaccine can offer benefit to selected children who are otitis media-prone. However, most clinical vaccine trials conducted in the 1980s failed to show a reduction in the overall incidence of AOM in these children (Table 7),[23-28] and few experts recommended routine use in the management of recurrent middle ear disease. The change in the antimicrobial susceptibility pattern for pneumococci, particularly a markedly increased resistance to amoxicillin, has reawakened interest in this potential pre-

Table 8: Tympanostomy Tubes for the Prevention of Recurrent AOM

Reference	Results
Gebhart (1981)[30]	Benefit demonstrated the prevention of recurrent AOM
Gonzalez et al (1986)[11]	No difference in AOM recurrence
Mandel et al (1989)[31]	Reduced recurrence of AOM
Casselbrant et al (1992)[17]	Reduced % time with AOM; no reduction in total episodes of AOM

ventive measure. Also, recent data suggest that the polysaccharide vaccine may be immunogenic in children as young as 8 months old,[29] questioning the requirement that children must be older than 2 years to be candidates for immunization. Once a conjugate pneumococcal vaccine becomes commercially available, the polysaccharide products likely will no longer be considered for use in any population of children or adults, analogous to the experience with the evolution of *H influenzae* type b vaccine preparations.

Tympanostomy Tubes

Only four studies have evaluated the efficacy of tympanostomy tube insertion in preventing recurrences of AOM (Table 8).[11,17,30,31] The first, published in 1981 by Gebhart,[30] demonstrated efficacy in the prevention of recurrent AOM, but patients were only followed for 6 months. Gonzalez et al[11] followed 65 children with previ-

Table 9: Adenoidectomy for the Prevention of Recurrent AOM

Study	Outcome
McKee (1963)[32]	Incidence of AOM reduced by 50% only during the first year post-surgery; no difference the second year
Mawson et al (1967)[33]	No reduction in recurrences of AOM during a 2-year follow-up
Roydhouse (1970)[34]	Reduction in incidence of AOM during the first year; no difference the second year. Reduced severity of AOM both years.

ous recurrent AOM, and concluded that effusions resolve more rapidly after tube placement, but that the overall incidence of AOM recurrence is not decreased. Only infants who had middle ear effusions at the time of enrollment were benefited. A larger study of tympanostomy tube placement versus no surgery was conducted by Casselbrant et al,[17] who randomized 264 children 7 to 35 months old who were otitis media-prone but who did not have OME at the time of entry into the study. The average rate of new episodes per child per year of either AOM or otorrhea was 1.08 in the control group and 1.02 in the tympanostomy tube group ($P=0.25$). However, the average proportion of time with OM of any type was 15% in controls, and 6.6% in those with tympanostomy tubes ($P<0.001$). The authors concluded that in this young age group, antibiotic chemoprophylaxis was the preferred first measure for preventing AOM recurrence, and that tympanostomy tubes should be reserved for children who fail medical prophylactic management.

Adenoidectomy

Adenoidectomy is a surgical intervention that has been recommended for children with recurrent AOM, but is generally reserved for patients who fail medical management and who have not benefited from tympanostomy tube insertion. This procedure has been used for the previous 70 years, but prospective clinical trials have only recently evaluated efficacy. The larger and better-designed clinical trials are included in Table 9.[32-34] Benefit, although afforded, is apparently limited to the first year after adenoidectomy, when the total incidence of AOM is reduced. One European study indicated that total AOM episodes were half of that in a control group,[32] and a similar study conducted in New Zealand showed a reduction to two thirds of the control incidence.[34] Although there is no consensus, otolaryngologists frequently recommend this procedure in more difficult cases where other therapy has failed (see Chapter 13).

References

1.   Rennels MB, Edwards KM, Keyserling HL, et al: Safety and immunogenicity of heptavalent pneumococcal vaccine conjugated to CRM_{197} in United States infants. *Pediatrics* 1998;101:604-611.

2.   Heikkinen T, Ruuskanen O, Waris M, et al: Influenza vaccination in the prevention of acute otitis media in children. *Am J Dis Child* 1991;145:445-448.

3.   Subramanian KN, Weisman LE, Rhodes T, et al: Safety, tolerance and pharmacokinetics of a humanized monoclonal antibody to respiratory syncytial virus in premature infants with bronchopulmonary dysplasia. MEDI-493 Study Group. *Pediatr Infect Dis J* 1998;17:110-115.

4.   Howie VM, Ploussard JH, Sloyer J: The "otitis-prone" condition. *Am J Dis Child* 1975;129:676-678.

5. Teele DW, Klein JO, Rosner B: Epidemiology of otitis media during the first seven years of life in children in greater Boston: a prospective, cohort study. *J Infect Dis* 1989;160:83-94.

6. Perrin JM, Charney E, MacWhinney JB Jr, et al: Sulfisoxazole as chemoprophylaxis for recurrent otitis media. A double-blind crossover study in pediatric practice. *N Engl J Med* 1974;291: 664-667.

7. Biedel CW: Modification of recurrent otitis media by short-term sulfonamide therapy. *Am J Dis Child* 1978;132:681-683.

8. Liston TE, Foshee WS, Pierson WD: Sulfisoxazole chemoprophylaxis for frequent otitis media. *Pediatrics* 1983;71:524-530.

9. Schuller DE: Prophylaxis of otitis media in asthmatic children. *Pediatr Infect Dis* 1983;2:280-283.

10. Varsano I, Volovitz B, Mimouni F: Sulfisoxazole prophylaxis of middle ear effusion and recurrent acute otitis media. *Am J Dis Child* 1985;139:632-635.

11. Gonzalez C, Arnold JE, Woody EA, et al: Prevention of recurrent acute otitis media: chemoprophylaxis versus tympanostomy tubes. *Laryngoscope* 1986;96:1330-1334.

12. Schwartz RH, Puglise J, Rodriguez WJ: Sulfamethoxazole prophylaxis in the otitis-prone child. *Arch Dis Child* 1982;57:590-593.

13. Lampe RM, Weir MR: Erythromycin prophylaxis for recurrent otitis media. *Clin Pediatr (Phila)* 1986;25:510-515.

14. Gray BM: Controlled trial of sulfamethoxazole-trimethoprim for the prevention of recurrent acute otitis media in young children. Proceedings of the 12th International Congress of Chemotherapy, Florence, Italy, July 19-24, 1981.

15. Dowell SF, Marcy SM, Phillips WR, et al: Otitis media—principles of judicious use of antimicrobial agents. *Pediatrics* 1998;101:S165-S171.

16. Principi N, Marchisio P, Massironi E, et al: Prophylaxis of recurrent acute otitis media and middle-ear effusion. Comparison of amoxicillin with sulfamethoxazole and trimethoprim. *Am J Dis Child* 1989;143:1414-1418.

17. Casselbrant ML, Kaleida PH, Rockette HE, et al: Efficacy of antimicrobial prophylaxis and of tympanostomy tube insertion for prevention of recurrent acute otitis media: results of a randomized clinical trial. *Pediatr Infect Dis J* 1992;11:278-286.

18. Berman S, Nuss R, Roark R, et al: Effectiveness of continuous vs. intermittent amoxicillin to prevent episodes of otitis media. *Pediatr Infect Dis J* 1992;11:63-67.

19. Maynard JE, Fleshman JK, Tschopp CF: Otitis media in Alaskan Eskimo children. Prospective evaluation of chemoprophylaxis. *JAMA* 1972;219:597-599.

20. Persico M, Podoshin L, Fradis M: Otitis media with effusion: a steroid and antibiotic therapeutic trial before surgery. *Ann Otol Rhinol Laryngol* 1978;87:191-196.

21. Uhari M, Kontiokari T, Niemela M: A novel use of xylitol sugar in preventing acute otitis media. *Pediatrics* 1998;102:879-884.

22. Chan KH, Bluestone CD: Lack of efficacy of middle-ear inflation: treatment of otitis media with effusion in children. *Otolaryngol Head Neck Surg* 1989;100:317-323.

23. Karma P, Luotonen J, Timonen M, et al: Efficacy of pneumococcal vaccination against recurrent otitis media. Preliminary results of a field trial in Finland. *Ann Otol Rhinol Laryngol Suppl* 1980;89:357-362.

24. Makela PH, Leinonen M, Pukander J, et al: A study of the pneumococcal vaccine in prevention of clinically acute attacks of recurrent otitis media. *Rev Infect Dis* 1981;3:S124-S132.

25. Sloyer JL Jr, Ploussard JH, Howie VM: Efficacy of pneumococcal polysaccharide vaccine in preventing acute otitis media in infants in Huntsville, Alabama. *Rev Infect Dis* 1981;3:S119-S123.

26. Teele DW, Pelton SI, Klein JO: Bacteriology of acute otitis media unresponsive to initial antimicrobial therapy. *J Pediatr* 1981;98:537-539.

27. Rosen C, Christensen P, Hovelius B, et al: Effect of pneumococcal vaccination on upper respiratory tract infections in children. Design of a follow-up study. *Scand J Infect Dis Suppl* 1983;39:39-44.

28. Howie VM, Ploussard JH, Sloyer JL, et al: Use of pneumococcal polysaccharide vaccine in preventing otitis media in infants: different results between racial groups. *Pediatrics* 1984;73:79-81.

29. Sorensen RU, Leiva LE, Giangrosso PA, et al: Response to a heptavalent conjugate *Streptococcus pneumoniae* vaccine in children with recurrent infections who are unresponsive to the polysaccharide vaccine. *Pediatr Infect Dis J* 1998;17:685-691.

30. Gebhart DE: Tympanostomy tubes in the otitis media prone child. *Laryngoscope* 1981;91:849-866.

31. Mandel EM, Rockette HE, Bluestone CD, et al: Myringotomy with and without tympanostomy tubes for chronic otitis media with effusion. *Arch Otolaryngol Head Neck Surg* 1989;115:1217-1224.

32. McKee WJ: A controlled study of the effects of tonsillectomy and adenoidectomy in children. *Br J Prev Soc Med* 1963;17:46-49.

33. Mawson SR, Adington R, Evans M: A controlled study evaluation of adeno-tonsillectomy in children. *J Laryngol Otol* 1967; 81:777-790.

34. Roydhouse N: A controlled study of adenotonsillectomy. *Arch Otolaryngol* 1970;92:611-616.

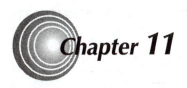

Chapter 11

Otitis Media With Effusion

Otitis media with effusion (OME) is defined as fluid in the middle ear without signs or symptoms of ear infection. This condition usually results from acute otitis media (AOM). After acute middle ear disease, effusions have been shown to persist for 1 month in approximately 40% of children, 2 months in 20%, and 3 months in 10%. OME is therefore the most frequent diagnosis for pediatric patients visiting U.S. physician offices, particularly infants and children under 3 years old.

The American Academy of Pediatrics, the American Academy of Family Physicians, and the American Academy of Otolaryngology—Head and Neck Surgery, with the review and approval of the Agency for Health Care Policy and Research of the U.S. Department of Health and Human Services, convened a panel of experts to develop a guideline on otitis media (OM) for providers and parents. Providers include primary care and specialist physicians, professional nurses and nurse practitioners, physician assistants, audiologists, speech-language pathologists, and child development specialists. Because the term *otitis media* encompasses a range of diseases, from acute to chronic and with or without symptoms, the Otitis Media Guideline Panel narrowed the topic to OME. Another expert panel is planned to address aspects of AOM.

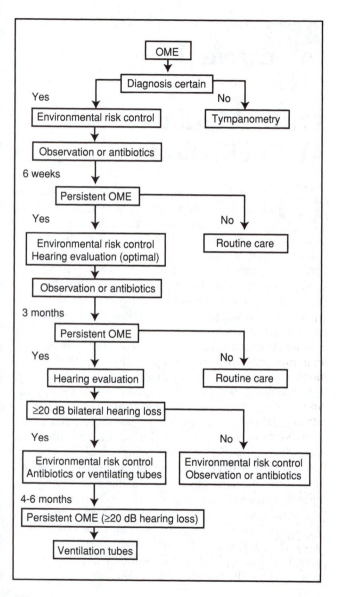

OME

Diagnosis certain

Yes → Environmental risk control

No → Tympanometry

Observation or antibiotics

6 weeks

Persistent OME

Yes → Environmental risk control / Hearing evaluation (optimal)

No → Routine care

Observation or antibiotics

3 months

Persistent OME

Yes → Hearing evaluation

No → Routine care

≥20 dB bilateral hearing loss

Yes → Environmental risk control / Antibiotics or ventilating tubes

No → Environmental risk control / Observation or antibiotics

4-6 months

Persistent OME (≥20 dB hearing loss)

Ventilation tubes

Figure 1: (a) OME is defined as fluid in the middle ear without signs or symptoms of infection. OME is not to be confused with AOM (inflammation of the middle ear with signs of infection). The guideline and this algorithm apply only to children with OME. This algorithm assumes follow-up intervals of 6 weeks.

(b) The algorithm applies only to children 1 to 3 years old with no craniofacial or neurologic abnormalities or sensory deficits (except as noted), and who are healthy except for OME. The guideline recommendations and algorithm do not apply if the child has any craniofacial or neurologic abnormality (eg, cleft palate, mental retardation) or sensory deficit (eg, decreased visual acuity or preexisting hearing deficit).

(c) The Otitis Media Guideline Panel found some evidence that pneumatic otoscopy is more accurate than otoscopy performed without the pneumatic test of eardrum mobility.

(d) Tympanometry may be used as confirmation of pneumatic otoscopy in the diagnosis of OME. Hearing evaluation is recommended for an otherwise healthy child who has had bilateral OME for 3 months; before 3 months, hearing evaluation is a clinical option.

(e) In most cases, OME resolves spontaneously within 3 months.

(f) The antibiotic drugs studied for treatment of OME were amoxicillin, amoxicillin/clavulanate, cefaclor, erythromycin, erythromycin/sulfisoxazole, sulfisoxazole, and trimethoprim/sulfamethoxazole.

(g) Exposure to cigarette smoke (passive smoking) has been shown to increase the risk of OME. For bottle-feeding versus breast-feeding and for child-care facility placement, associations were found with OME, but evidence available to the panel did not show decreased incidence of OME with breast-feeding or with removal from child-care facilities.

(h) The recommendation against tonsillectomy is based on the lack of added benefit of tonsillectomy when (continued on next page)

173

Figure 1 (continued from previous page):
combined with adenoidectomy to treat OME in older children. Tonsillectomy and adenoidectomy may be appropriate for reasons other than OME.
(i) The panel found evidence that decongestants and antihistamines are ineffective treatments for OME.
(j) Meta-analysis failed to show a significant benefit for corticosteroids without antibiotic medications in treating OME in children.

Recommendations and options developed by this guideline panel for the diagnosis and management of OME in otherwise healthy young children are summarized below and in Figure 1. This document addressed the management of OME in children ages 1 to 3 years with no cranial, facial, or neurologic abnormalities or sensory deficits. These children are assumed to be healthy except for OME.

Natural History

Longitudinal studies of OME show spontaneous resolution of the condition in more than half of children within 3 months of development of the effusion. After 3 months, the rate of spontaneous resolution remains constant, so that only a small percentage of children experience OME lasting 1 year or longer. In most children, episodes of OME do not persist beyond early childhood. The likelihood that middle ear fluid will resolve by itself underlies the recommendations for management of OME.

Environmental Risk Factors

Scientific evidence showed that the following environmental factors may increase the risk of AOM or OME:
• Bottle-feeding rather than breast-feeding infants
• Passive smoking
• Group child-care facility attendance
Because the guideline recommendations target children who are beyond the age when breast-feeding ver-

sus bottle-feeding is an issue, this risk factor was not considered at length.

Passive smoking (exposure to another's tobacco smoke) is associated with a higher risk of OME. Although there is no proof that stopping passive smoking helps prevent middle ear fluid, there are many health reasons for not exposing persons of any age to tobacco smoke. Therefore, clinicians should advise parents of the benefits of decreasing children's exposure to tobacco smoke.

Studies of OME in children cared for at home compared to those in group child-care facilities found that children in group child-care facilities have a slightly higher relative risk of OME (less than 2.0). Research did not show whether removing the child from the group child-care facility helped prevent OME.

Highlights of Patient Management

Congenital or early-onset hearing impairment is a widely accepted risk factor for impaired speech and language development. In general, earlier onset and increased severity of the hearing problem correlates with worse effects on speech and language development. Because OME is often associated with a mild to moderate hearing loss, most clinicians have been eager to treat the condition to restore hearing to normal, and thus prevent any long-term problems.

Studies of the effects of OME on hearing have varied in design, and have examined several aspects of hearing and communication skills. Because of these differences, the results cannot be combined to provide a clear picture of the relationship between OME and hearing. Also, it is uncertain whether changes in hearing caused by middle ear fluid have any long-term effects on development. Evidence of dysfunctions mediated by OME that have persisted into later childhood, despite resolution of the middle ear fluid and a return to normal hearing, would provide a compelling argument for early, decisive intervention. However, no consistent, reliable evidence suggests that OME has such long-term effects on language or learning.

The following recommendations for managing OME are tempered by the failure to find rigorous, methodologically sound research to support the theory that untreated OME results in speech and language delays or deficits.

Diagnosis and Hearing Evaluation

(1) *Suspect OME in young children.* Most children have at least one episode of OME before entering school. OME may be identified after an episode of AOM, or it may be an incidental finding. Symptoms may include discomfort or behavior changes.

(2) *Use pneumatic otoscopy to assess middle ear status.* Pneumatic otoscopy is recommended for assessment of the middle ear because it combines visualization of the tympanic membrane mobility (otoscopy) with a test of membrane mobility (pneumatic otoscopy). When pneumatic otoscopy is performed by an experienced examiner, the accuracy of diagnosis of OME may be between 70% and 79%.

(3) *Tympanometry may be performed to confirm suspected OME.* Tympanometry provides an indirect measure of tympanic membrane compliance and an estimate of middle ear air pressure. The positive predictive value of an abnormal (type B, flat) tympanogram is between 49% and 99%; ie, as few as half of ears with abnormal tympanograms may have OME. The negative predictive value of this test is better: most middle ears with normal tympanograms are actually normal. Because the strengths of tympanometry (a quantitative measure of tympanic membrane mobility) and pneumatic otoscopy (visualization of many abnormalities of the eardrum and ear canal that can skew the results of tympanometry) offset the weaknesses of each, the two tests together improve the accuracy of diagnosis. Acoustic reflectometry has not been studied well enough to yield a

Table 1: Benefits of Treating Otitis Media With Effusion

Intervention	Benefits
Observation	Base case
Antibiotics	Improved clearance of effusion at 1 month or less, 14% (95% confidence interval 3.6%, 24.2%; possible reduction in future infections)
Antibiotics plus corticosteroids	Possible improved clearance at 1 month, 25.1% (95% confidence interval -1.3%, 49.9%; possible reduction in future infections)
Corticosteroids alone	Possible improved clearance at 1 month, 4.5% (95% confidence interval -11.7%, 20.6%)
Antihistamine/ decongestant	Same as base case
Myringotomy with tubes	Immediate clearance of effusion in all children; improved hearing
Adenoidectomy	Benefits for young children have not been established
Tonsillectomy	Same as base case

recommendation for or against its use to diagnose OME. Also, no recommendation is made about the use of tuning fork tests to screen for or diagnose OME, except that they are inappropriate in the youngest children.

(4) *A child who has had fluid in both middle ears for a total of 3 months should undergo hearing evaluation. Be-*

Table 2: Adverse Effects of Treating Otitis Media With Effusion

Intervention	Benefits
Observation	Base case
Antibiotics	Nausea, vomiting, diarrhea (2% to 32% depending on dose and antibiotic); cutaneous reaction (≤5%); numerous rare organ system effects, including very rare fatalities; cost; possible development of resistant strains of bacteria
Antibiotics plus corticosteroids	Same as antibiotics and corticosteroids separately
Corticosteroids alone	Possible exacerbation of varicella; long-term complications not established for low doses; cost
Antihistamine/decongestant	Drowsiness; excitability; cost
Myringotomy with tubes	Invasive procedure; anesthesia risk; cost; tympanosclerosis; otorrhea; possible restrictions on swimming
Adenoidectomy	Invasive procedure; anesthesia risk; cost
Tonsillectomy	Invasive procedure; anesthesia risk; cost

fore 3 months of effusion, hearing evaluation is an option. A change in hearing threshold is both a clinical outcome and a possible indicator of the presence of OME. Methods to determine a child's hearing acuity vary, depending on available resources and the child's willingness and ability to participate in testing. Optimally, air and bone conduction thresholds can be established for 500, 1,000, 2,000, and 4,000 Hz, and an air-conduction pure tone average can be calculated. This result should be verified by obtaining a measure of speech sensitivity.

Determinations of speech reception threshold or speech awareness threshold alone may be used if the child cannot cooperate in pure tone testing. If none of the test techniques is available or tolerated, the examiner should use his or her best judgment of adequacy of hearing. In these cases, the health-care provider should be aware of whether the child is achieving appropriate developmental milestones for verbal communication.

Although hearing evaluation may be difficult to perform in young children, evaluation is recommended after bilateral OME has been present for 3 months, because of the strong belief that surgery is not indicated unless OME is causing hearing impairment (defined as equal to or worse than 20 dB hearing threshold level in the better-hearing ear).

(5) *Observation or antibiotic therapy are treatment options for children with effusion that has been present less than 4 to 6 months, and at any time for children without a 20-dB hearing threshold level or worse in the better-hearing ear.* Most cases of OME resolve spontaneously. Meta-analysis of controlled studies showed a 14% increase in the resolution rate when antibiotics were given. Length of treatment in these studies was typically 10 days.

The most common adverse effects of antibiotic therapy are gastrointestinal. Dermatologic reactions may occur in 3% to 5% of cases; severe anaphylactic reactions are much rarer. Severe hematologic, cardiovascular, central nervous system, endocrine, renal, hepatic, and respiratory adverse effects are rarer still. The potential for the development of microbial resistance is always present with antibiotics.

(6) *For a child who has had bilateral effusion for a total of 3 months and who has a bilateral hearing deficiency (defined as a 20-dB hearing threshold level or worse in the better-hearing ear), bilateral myringotomy with tube insertion becomes an additional treatment option. Placement of tympanostomy tubes is recommended after a total of 4 to 6 months of bilateral effusion with a bilateral hearing deficit.* The principal benefits of myringotomy with insertion of tympanostomy tubes are the restoration of hearing to the pre-effusion threshold and clearance of the fluid and possible feeling of pressure. While patent and in place, tubes may prevent further accumulation of fluid in the middle ear. Although evidence is insufficient to prove that OME has long-term deleterious effects, concern about the possibility of such effects led the expert panel to recommend surgery. A myriad of tube designs are available, most constructed from plastic or metal. Data comparing outcomes with tubes of various designs are sparse; thus, the panel assumed no notable differences among available tympanostomy tubes.

Insertion of tympanostomy tubes is performed under general anesthesia in young children. Calculation of the risks for two specific complications of myringotomy with tympanostomy tube insertion showed that tympanosclerosis might occur after this procedure in 51%, and postoperative otorrhea in 13% of children.

A number of treatments are not recommended for OME in an otherwise healthy child between ages 1 and 3 years:
• *Corticosteroids* are not recommended to treat OME in a child of any age because of limited scientific evidence that this treatment is effective, and because of the opinion of many experts that the possible adverse effects (eg, agitation, behavior change, and more serious problems such as disseminated varicella in children exposed to this virus within the month before therapy) outweigh possible benefits.
• *Antihistamine/decongestant therapy* is not recommended for treatment of OME in a child of any age, be-

cause review of the literature showed that these agents are not effective for this condition, either separately or together.

• *Adenoidectomy* is not an appropriate treatment for uncomplicated middle ear effusion in a child younger than 4 years old when adenoid pathology is not present, based on the lack of scientific evidence. Potential harms for children of all ages include the risks of general anesthesia and the possibility of excessive postoperative bleeding.

• *Tonsillectomy, either alone or with adenoidectomy*, has not been found effective for treatment of OME.

• *The association between allergy and OME* was not clear from available evidence. Thus, although close anatomic relationships between the nasopharynx, eustachian tube, and middle ear have led many experts to suggest a role for allergy management in treating OME, no recommendation was made for or against such treatment.

• *Evidence for other therapies for the treatment of OME* was sought, but no reports of chiropractic, holistic, naturopathic, traditional/indigenous, homeopathic, or other treatments contained information obtained in randomized controlled studies. Therefore, no recommendation was made about such other therapies for the treatment of OME in children.

Treatment Outcomes

Table 1 summarizes the benefits and Table 2 outlines the adverse consequences, of management interventions for OME.

Selected Readings

Stool SE, Berg AO, Berman S, et al: Managing otitis media with effusion in young children. Quick Reference Guide for Clinicians. Rockville, MD, Agency for Health Care Policy and Research. Public Health Service, U.S. Department of Health and Human Services, July 1994. AHCPR Publication 94-0623.

Black N: The aetiology of glue ear—a case-control study. *Int J Pediatr Otorhinolaryngol* 1985;9:121-133.

Cantekin EI, Mandel EM, Bluestone CD, et al: Lack of efficacy of a decongestant-antihistamine combination for otitis media with effusion ("secretory" otitis media) in children. Results of a double-blind, randomized trial. *N Engl J Med* 1983;308:297-301.

Casselbrant ML, Brostoff LM, Cantekin EI, et al: Otitis media with effusion in preschool children. *Laryngoscope* 1985;95:428-436.

Etzel RA, Pattishall EN, Haley NJ, et al: Passive smoking and middle ear effusion among children in day care. *Pediatrics* 1992;90:228-232.

Friel-Patti S, Finitzo T: Language learning in a prospective study of otitis media with effusion in the first two years of life. *J Speech Hear Res* 1990;33:188-194.

Maw AR: Development of tympanosclerosis in children with otitis media with effusion and ventilation tubes. *J Laryngol Otol* 1991;105:614-617.

Rosenfeld RM, Mandel EM, Bluestone CD: Systemic steroids for otitis media with effusion in children. *Arch Otolaryngol Head Neck Surg* 1991;117:984-989.

Rosenfeld RM, Post JC: Meta-analysis of antibiotics for the treatment of otitis media with effusion. *Otolaryngol Head Neck Surg* 1992;106:378-386.

Teele DW, Klein JO, Rosner B, et al: Middle ear disease and the practice of pediatrics. Burden during the first five years of life. *JAMA* 1983;249:1026-1029.

Teele DW, Klein JO, Rosner BA: Otitis media with effusion during the first three years of life and development of speech and language. *Pediatrics* 1984;74:282-287.

Toner JG, Mains B: Pneumatic otoscopy and tympanometry in the detection of middle ear effusion. *Clin Otolaryngol* 1990;15:121-123.

Williams RL, Chalmers TC, Stange KC, et al: Use of antibiotics in preventing recurrent acute otitis media and in treating otitis media with effusion. A meta-analytic attempt to resolve the brouhaha. *JAMA* 1993;270:1344-1351.

Zielhuis GA, Straatman H, Rach GH, et al: Analysis and presentation of data on the natural course of otitis media with effusion in children. *Int J Epidemiol* 1990;19:1037-1044.

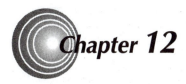

Chapter 12

Chronic Otitis Media

Chronic otitis media refers to a permanent perforation of the tympanic membrane (TM) with or without active infection and drainage. The presence or absence of chronic otorrhea and inflammation determines whether a chronic perforation is *dry* (free of infection) or *wet* (without otorrhea). When a perforation includes infection and drainage, it is classified as chronic suppurative otitis media (CSOM). CSOM may occur with or without cholesteatoma, and is believed to represent a chronic stage of acute otitis media (AOM).[1] This chapter describes chronic perforations and CSOM without cholesteatoma; CSOM with cholesteatoma is examined in Chapter 15.

Chronic Perforations

Perforations of the TM, which occur for a variety of reasons, generally persist secondary to eustachian tube (ET) dysfunction. Chronic perforations in children most often occur secondary to tympanostomy tubes or to acute infections. Perforations secondary to AOM occur when the purulence under pressure ruptures the TM, most often the pars tensa. Some evidence suggests that spontaneous perforations may prevent further otitis media (OM)-related complications. While these acute perforations generally heal within a few weeks, occasionally the perforation persists and the ear continues to drain. When the perforation persists, a rim of scar forms (fusion of the undersurface and surface of the TM) circumferentially

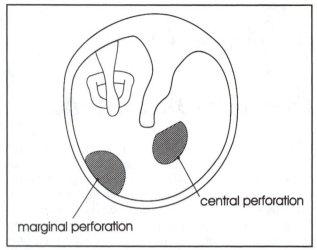

central perforation

marginal perforation

Figure 1: *Central perforations have at least a small border of tympanic membrane around all the edges. Marginal perforations extend to the annulus in at least one portion of the perforation.*

around the edges, preventing healing. American Indians and Eskimos have a high predisposition to spontaneous perforations. It is difficult to determine whether a draining perforation is secondary to poor ET function or to chronic water contamination in an active bather.

Perforations are described by their size and location. Size is determined by either the percentage of TM loss (eg, 10%) or as small, medium, or large. Location is described as either central or marginal. Central perforations have at least a small border of TM around all the edges; marginal perforations extend to the annulus in at least one portion of the perforation (Figure 1).

The position of the perforation has clinical implications. Marginal perforations are more difficult to repair and have a greater risk of external canal skin growing into the middle ear, ie, predisposition to cholesteatoma formation. An extremely atelectatic retraction pocket may resemble (and therefore be difficult to differentiate from) a perforation. Differentiation between a perforation and retraction can usually be determined by pneumatic insufflation or by spraying boric acid onto the area. Boric acid sprayed into a perforation dissolves in the moist middle ear mucosa; in a true retraction pocket, which is dry epithelium, the boric acid remains a powder.

Treatment: Chronic Perforations

The goals of surgical treatment are to restore TM integrity and to prevent recurrent middle ear infection. The surgical removal of ventilation tubes results in an iatrogenic perforation that often heals. A study comparing the Gelfoam®/Gelfilm® patching of these perforations after the surgical removal of ventilation tubes in pediatric patients demonstrated a significant difference in the rate of persistent TM perforation: 10.3% without patching versus 4.5% with patching.[2]

Clinicians continue to debate when to surgically repair a perforation to avoid continued ET dysfunction in this population. A small chronic perforation provides function, ventilation, and drainage, similar to a tympanostomy tube. A chronic perforation also leaves the middle ear vulnerable to chronic environmental contamination. Most physicians delay repair of perforations until ET function is optimized. It may be difficult to differentiate whether a draining perforation is secondary to poor ET function or to chronic water contamination in an active bather. At least 3 months of observation should be allowed for spontaneous closure before perforation repair.

Studies examining factors related to tympanoplasty outcomes in children with post-tympanostomy tube perforations found graft success of 94.6% and reperforations occurring in 5.4% during an average follow-up of 16.8 months.[3] These studies also indicate that surgical outcome

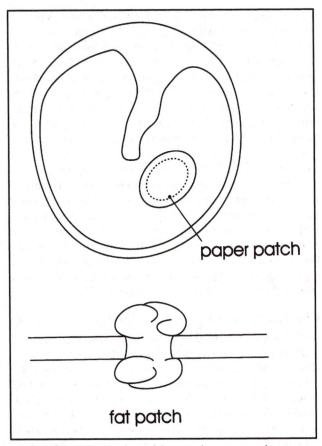

Figure 2: *Paper patch and fat patch myringoplasty.*

is not influenced by age, technique, or size or position of the perforation. A similar study performed at the House Ear Clinic[4] examined children of different age groups: 7 to 8 years, 9 to 12 years, and 13 to 19 years, and their retrospective tympanoplasty success rates. Interestingly, they found no difference in outcome among the four age groups, with an intact graft in 92.5% of ears and a postoperative air-bone gap of less than 25 dB in 84% of ears.

The size of the TM perforation determines the repair approach. The *paper patch*, a straightforward outpatient procedure, may be performed on smaller central perforations. This procedure involves freshening the edges with trichloroacetic acid and patching the perforation with cigarette paper (Figure 2). For slightly larger perforations, a fat myringoplasty can be performed, which also involves freshening the edges. A small amount of fat harvested from the lobule is used to plug the perforation (Figure 2).

A formal tympanoplasty is performed when the perforation is large or marginal. Audiometric evaluation should be performed before otologic surgery. Approach to the perforation may be either postauricular or transcanal. *Rimming* of the perforation must be performed before repair because failure to remove the scar tissue prevents healing. A temporalis fascia graft is harvested postauricularly and placed medial to the TM perforation.

Chronic Suppurative Otitis Media

CSOM is believed to result from inadequately treated AOM. It is characterized by painless otorrhea from a chronic TM perforation. In chronic ear disease, the process is often slow, progressive, and unrelenting, compared to an acute infection, which has a rapid onset that often results in swift resolution. The chronic, insidious nature of the disease may lead to destructive complications. Chronic mastoiditis is often an important component of CSOM.

Pathologic Changes

Chronic inflammation can cause permanent changes in the middle ear mucosa with resultant granulation tissue. The granulation tissue produces an osteitis, bony destruction, and secondary complications. Chronic inflammatory cells, including mononuclear and polymorphonuclear leukocytes, infiltrate the middle ear mucosa. This results in inflammation and edema, leading to chronic obstruction and polyp formation. The chronic state of inflammation may have quiescent periods, but these are often interrupted by periods of active drainage. These inflammatory changes are often irreversible unless treated quickly (within 6 weeks) and aggressively.

Predisposing Factors

In a child with a chronically draining ear, the most common predisposing factor is ET dysfunction. ET function usually matures by age 6. Adenoid hypertrophy, especially in conjunction with a contralateral serous OM, may result in a chronically draining ear. The status of the contralateral ear is an important indicator of ET function. Nasal foreign bodies should also be included in the differential diagnosis in a child with a chronically draining ear. The author has treated a child with CSOM whose symptoms resolved almost immediately after the identification and removal of a piece of sponge in the nasopharynx. Certain ethnic groups, such as American Indians and Eskimos, are predisposed to chronically draining ears. A chronically draining ear may also indicate a systemic disease: metabolic, autoimmune, or vascular. Neoplastic processes, such as eosinophilic granuloma, may also present as CSOM.

Office Treatment

Before surgical intervention, all attempts should be made to obtain a *dry* ear. This is attainable in CSOM without cholesteatoma, but is more elusive in CSOM with cholesteatoma. Great care must be taken to prevent the otorrhea from draining into the external ear and neck, because this may result in significant skin excoriation and dermatitis. Obtaining a dry ear requires aggressive office débridement and appropriate topical and systemic antimicrobial therapy. Topical antimicrobial preparations containing neomycin/polymyxin or an aminoglycoside (eg,

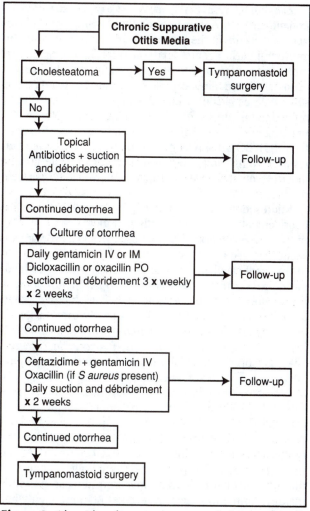

Figure 3: Algorithm for management of chronic suppurative otitis media (CSOM), including option for once-daily gentamicin outpatient therapy and indications for tympanomastoid surgery.

gentamicin [Garamycin®]), as well as a corticosteroid component, are effective in treating the draining ear. Controversy exists about the potential ototoxicity of these topical therapeutic agents. Experimental data demonstrate ototoxicity secondary to otic drops, although this has not been confirmed clinically. The literature has documented several cases of sensorineural hearing loss believed to be related to otic drops in patients with CSOM.[5] Recent development of a topical fluoroquinolone (ciprofloxacin, Cipro® HC Otic) shows great promise. Prospective studies examining topical ciprofloxacin demonstrate it to be more effective than topical gentamicin for the treatment of chronic OM.[6]

Microscopic visualization is quite helpful during office débridement; an otoscope with a surgical head may also provide visualization. The microscope allows for precise suctioning and assessment of the TM. Careful cleaning of the external canal and middle ear cleft allows for both adequate assessment and access for topical antibiotics. A mixed flora, including aerobic and anaerobic pathogens, are commonly cultured, most frequently gram-negative organisms. *Pseudomonas aeruginosa* is most common, followed by *Staphylococcus aureus*, *Escherichia coli*, and anaerobic organisms. Culturing of the otorrhea is not usually necessary unless no response results from the empiric treatment. In rare resistant cases, intravenous antibiotics may be used. Avoidance of water exposure is integral to medical therapy.

In about 10% of patients, persistent otorrhea occurs after tympanostomy tubes are inserted. This occurs more often in younger children. Initial therapy involves suctioning the purulent debris and administering topical antibiotic therapy. Oral antibiotics are added to the regimen when there is no response to topical therapy. In rare intractable cases, intravenous antibiotics are given that cover the commonly cultured *Pseudomonas* species. When there is no response to this intensive therapy, myringotomy tube removal is considered; very rarely, mastoidectomy and middle ear exploration are performed.

Surgical Intervention: CSOM

The goals of surgical intervention in CSOM are to provide a dry, safe ear and to restore function (ie, hearing). Some experts recommend tympanoplasty alone to prevent recurrence, since reinfection is caused by nasopharyngeal reflux of organisms or water penetration from the external canal. Others assert that CSOM requires mastoidectomy in conjunction with tympanoplasty to eliminate the nidus of chronic infection. A recent retrospective study examined this question[7] by comparing tympanoplasty without mastoidectomy to tympanoplasty with mastoidectomy in patients with CSOM without cholesteatoma. Some were actively draining, while others were dry at surgery. No statistically significant differences were found between dry and discharging ears, type of surgical intervention, or graft success and final functional hearing. Despite this finding, most otolaryngologists continue to perform mastoidectomy for a chronically draining ear.

Sequelae

The destructive effects of CSOM result from a slow, insidious process. Children with chronic perforations and CSOM most often present with conductive hearing loss. The severity of the loss depends on the position and size of the perforation and the status of the ossicular chain and inner ear. Ossicular erosion or disarticulation should be considered if the conductive loss is greater than 30 dB. Hearing may improve during active drainage. A sensorineural hearing loss may occur when a labyrinthine or cochlear fistula is present.

Complications of CSOM without cholesteatoma are similar to those of CSOM with cholesteatoma (Chapter 16). Facial nerve paresis may occur when granulation tissue compresses the facial nerve. Surgical removal of the granulation tissue with proximal and distal decompression usually results in full recovery. Meningitis secondary to CSOM usually results from direct pathogen spread or through the round or oval window. Intensive antibiotic therapy directed against common CSOM organisms, *P aeruginosa* and *S aureus*, is appropriate. The diseased tissue should be surgically removed when the patient is stable and able to tolerate general anesthesia.

References

1. Bluestone CD: Epidemiology and pathogenesis of chronic suppurative otitis media: implications for prevention and treatment. *Int J Pediatr Otorhinolaryngol* 1998;42:207-223.

2. Hekkenberg RJ, Smitheringale AJ: Gelfoam/Gelfilm patching following the removal of ventilation tubes. *J Otolaryngol* 1995; 24:362-363.

3. Te GO, Rizer FM, Schuring AG: Pediatric tympanoplasty of iatrogenic perforations from ventilation tube therapy. *Am J Otol* 1998;19:301-305.

4. Chandrasekhar SS, House JW, Devgan U: Pediatric tympanoplasty. A 10-year experience. *Arch Otolaryngol Head Neck Surg* 1995;121:873-878.

5. Linder TE, Zwicky S, Brandle P: Ototoxicity of ear drops: a clinical perspective. *Am J Otol* 1995;16:653-657.

6. Tutkun A, Ozagar A, Koc A, et al: Treatment of chronic ear disease. Topical ciprofloxacin vs topical gentamicin. *Arch Otolaryngol Head Neck Surg* 1995;121:1414-1416.

7. Balyan FR, Celikkanat S, Aslan A, et al: Mastoidectomy in noncholesteatomatous chronic suppurative otitis media: is it necessary? *Otolaryngol Head Neck Surg* 1997;117:592-595.

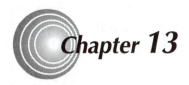

Chapter 13

Surgical Therapy in Otitis Media

Medical therapy is the first-line treatment in acute otitis media (AOM) and otitis media with effusion (OME). Surgical therapy is considered only after intensive medical therapy has failed. Surgery is intended to address both the underlying pathophysiology (ie, poor ventilation) and the sequelae (eg, hearing loss, chronic illness). Three surgical procedures are used to treat otitis media (OM): tympanocentesis, tympanostomy tube insertion, and adenoidectomy.

Tympanocentesis

Tympanocentesis (diagnostic aspiration) may be quite helpful in the diagnostic and therapeutic management of a child with AOM. Tympanocentesis, once widely performed, has declined significantly in the era of antibiotics. With the increase in resistant organisms, interest in this procedure has been broadening. Indications for tympanocentesis include use in a healthy child who is not responding to conventional antibiotics or who is suspected of having resistant organisms, an immunosuppressed child or newborn infant with OM and sepsis, and a child in unusually severe pain (Table 1). When suppurative and nonsuppurative complications occur in association with OM and both bacterial diagnosis and middle ear drainage are desired, a wide myringotomy may be performed. Gram stain and culture of the aspirated fluid allows for culture-

Table 1: Indications for Tympanocentesis in Otitis Media

- Not responsive to conventional antibiotics
- Suspect resistant organisms
- Immunosuppressive child
- Newborn infant
- Unusually severe pain
- Complication related to otitis media

directed antibiotic therapy. Although tympanocentesis may aid in pain relief, it does not appear to accelerate resolution of the infection or effusion.

Most clinicians do not use anesthesia when performing tympanocentesis, especially in neonates. The acute inflammation generally makes obtaining an adequate anesthetic block difficult, especially considering the brevity of the procedure. Topical anesthetics, placed on the tympanic membrane and external auditory canal, have recently been considered. A study comparing the use of EMLA® cream (lidocaine and prilocaine) and Bonain's solution (equal amounts of cocaine hydrochloride, menthol, and phenol) found Bonain's solution significantly more effective.[1]

The laser-assisted myringotomy is the most recent development. This device produces a myringotomy that is maintained for up to 6 weeks. The proponents of laser-assisted myringotomy argue that increasing bacterial resistance requires additional methods of treatment. They think that this method may even be a primary treatment of AOM.

Procedure

Once the child is immobilized (as described in Chapter 1), the tympanic membrane is visualized with either

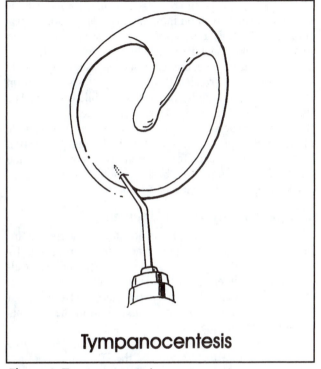

Tympanocentesis

Figure 1: Tympanocentesis.

an otologic microscope or an otoscope with a surgical head. The external auditory canal is initially cleared of cerumen and debris after the external canal is sterilized with alcohol or an iodine-containing solution. The intended area for tympanocentesis is the inferior quadrants; the posterior-superior quadrant poses undue risk to the ossicular chain. An Alden-Senturi® trap or 'tymp-tap' with an 18-gauge needle, or simply a bent 21-gauge needle attached to a 3-mL syringe, is used to aspirate the middle ear fluid (Figure 1). The fluid is sent in appropriate microbial vials to the laboratory.

When a wide myringotomy is performed for indications such as mastoiditis or an intracranial complication, a myringotomy knife is used to make an incision large enough to allow for adequate drainage and ventilation. In this procedure, sedation or general anesthesia is usually required.

Complications related to tympanocentesis are rare in experienced hands with a properly immobilized child. The tympanic membrane and external canal are vulnerable to the trauma associated with a child's sudden jerks. A wide myringotomy poses greater risks, including perforation and chronic otorrhea. Other extremely rare risks include puncture of the jugular bulb, severing the facial nerve, or dislocating the ossicular chain.

Tympanostomy Tube Placement

Tympanostomy tube (TT) placement is the most common surgical procedure performed on children. The TT works where the eustachian tube (ET) has failed. It allows for both ventilation and drainage of the middle ear. It does not protect, however, and leaves the middle ear vulnerable to water and contaminants from the external canal and environment.

Because OM is most commonly related to ET dysfunction, the TT in effect 'bypasses' the ET. It does not address the multifactorial nature of OM, including underlying immunodeficiency or allergy. Despite the frequency of TT placement, it remains controversial. Debate ranges from a belief that it is an overused and unnecessary procedure, to support as a procedure that both restores hearing and decreases morbidity.

TT placement does not correct the underlying pathology (ie, ET dysfunction); it merely 'bypasses' it. This is illustrated in that the recurrence of middle ear effusion mirrors the time of TT extrusion. The type of tube affects the retention time: a larger-bore TT with a T-shape lasts longer (Figure 2). However, these tubes also have a higher incidence of perforation.

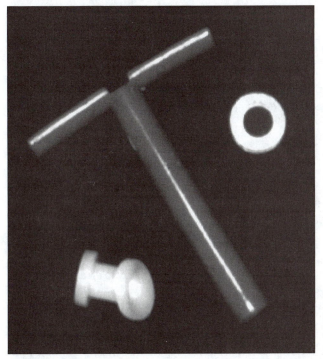

Figure 2: Tympanostomy tube types.

Indications for TT placement include OME, recurrent OM, significant retraction, and suppurative complications (Table 2). In 1994, the Agency for Health Care Policy and Research (AHCPR) presented the Clinical Practice Guidelines for Otitis Media with Effusion.[2] These include an algorithm for treating otherwise healthy children with OME between ages 1 and 3. TT placement was recommended in children who, after appropriate medical treatment, had bilateral effusions longer than 3 months with associated hearing loss. Although not addressed by the AHCPR, TT placement should also be considered in children with persistent middle ear effusion without hearing

Table 2: Indications for Tympanostomy Tube Placement

- Recurrent otitis media (ROM)
- Otitis media with effusion (OME)
- OME or ROM with
  - Craniofacial anomalies (eg, cleft palate)
  - Down syndrome
- Tympanic membrane abnormalities, including severe atelectasis or retraction pocket
- Suppurative complication

loss, as well as those with persistent unilateral effusion (>6 months). Children with thick, mucoid fluid rather than scanty serous effusions are less likely to clear their middle ear effusions.

A recent article examined adherence to the AHCPR guidelines. The results indicated that delayed referral occurred in 34% of patients, while 25% of patients were referred early.[3] The average duration of effusion in patients with OME was 5.2 months; the duration of recurrent AOM immediately before referral was 9.3 months. In the OME group, 47% of the children had a history of recurrent chronic OME spanning an average of 22.7 months. On referral, hearing loss was discovered in 92% of patients, and, in 69%, the tympanogram was flat. The complication and sequelae rate was 49.1%; speech delay was most common at 16.9%.

Most physicians use the following criteria for TT placement: a minimum of 4 episodes of recurrent OM in a 6-month period after the failure of both antimicrobial therapy and chemoprophylaxis. Although episodes of OM in this group respond to medical therapy and effusions clear promptly, the morbidity associated with the frequency and

Table 3: Recommendations for Otolaryngologic Referral

- Recurrent otitis media despite intensive medical therapy
- Otitis media with effusion for >3 months
- Speech or language delay
- Hearing loss ≥20 dB
- Suppurative or nonsuppurative complications
- Secondary complications of OM (atelectasis, retraction pocket, cholesteatoma)

the severity of the illness (fever and otalgia), and the intermittent decrease in hearing, often make TT an essential next step (Table 3). A recent outcome study evaluating changes in health-related quality of life for children with OM demonstrated significant improvement in quality of life after TT.[4]

Other less common indications for TT placement include atelectasis and retraction pockets of the tympanic membrane, or an OM-related complication. As described in Chapter 12, the tympanic membrane may become flaccid and retracted secondary to continued negative middle ear pressure. Severe retraction may result in ossicular erosion and conductive hearing loss, or evolve into a cholesteatoma. TT insertion may reequilibrate middle ear pressure and return the tympanic membrane to its original position. End-stage retractions do not typically respond to TT placement. Children who have sustained an OM-related complication generally require TT insertion to both identify the causative organism and provide middle ear ventilation. TT insertion may be quite challenging in patients with mastoiditis because of an extremely inflamed and edematous external canal and tympanic membrane.

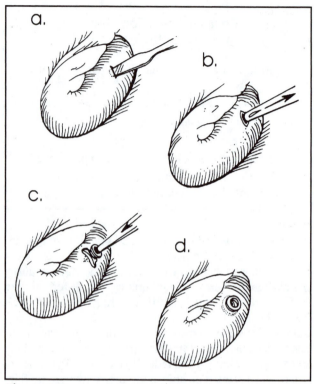

Figure 3: Tympanostomy tube placement.

OME also significantly affects balance and coordination skills in children. These skills improve after TT insertion, compared with controls.[5]

Procedure

TT placement is typically performed with masked general anesthesia under microscopic visualization. Initially, the external auditory canal is cleared of cerumen and the tympanic membrane is visualized. A myringotomy knife is used to make an incision in the drum anterior-inferior or posterior-inferior quadrants (Figure 3). Care is taken to avoid the posterior-superior quadrant because of the risk of ossicular disruption, both immediate and with future tube migration.

Potential complications include perforation, chronic otorrhea, granulation tissue, and cholesteatoma. Water precautions are important because the TT leaves the middle ear vulnerable, an important cause of chronic drainage. In addition, it is extremely important that the patient be followed until the TT extrudes. Cholesteatoma formation may rarely occur if not monitored closely.

Adenoidectomy

The adenoids (pharyngeal tonsils) are an aggregate of lymphoid tissue on the posterior and superior wall of the nasopharynx. Together with the lingual tonsils and palatine tonsils, they form a ring of lymphoid tissue known as Waldeyer's ring. The adenoids appear to be involved in regulating secretory immunity, and are predominantly B-cell organs. The adenoids enlarge during early childhood in response to antigenic challenges, sometimes resulting in nasal obstruction. After the fifth year of life, the adenoids atrophy while the nasopharynx enlarges, improving nasal breathing. The eustachian tubes are just lateral to this mass of tissue. Their function is affected both directly (mass effect) and indirectly (bacterial colonization) by the adenoid pad.

Adenoidectomy in the treatment of OM remains controversial.[6] It is not considered effective, according to the AHCPR, for 'uncomplicated middle ear effusion' in children under 4 years old. Adenoidectomy is generally used as an adjunct when TT has failed, usually in an older age group, rather than as a primary surgical treatment. Studies have demonstrated benefit of adenoidectomy in children between 4 and 8 years old. Interestingly, three clinical studies have demonstrated that the success of adenoidectomy does not seem to be correlated with ade-

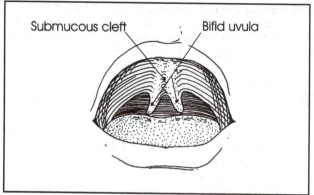

Figure 4: *Submucous cleft.*

noid size. The presence of bacterial colonization of the adenoids appears to be the source of inoculation in recurrent OM. In a recent study, bacteriologic analysis of adenoids demonstrated an elevated colonization rate of middle ear pathogens in children with present or history of ear disease, compared with children with only adenoid hypertrophy. The predominant pathogens were nontypeable *Haemophilus influenzae, Streptococcus pneumoniae*, and *Moraxella catarrhalis*. In addition, studies have demonstrated no difference in outcome (ie, hearing and recurrence of OM) between TT placement and adenoidectomy with myringotomy. While TT insertion merely 'bypasses' the pathology in OM, adenoidectomy theoretically addresses the underlying pathology, whether it is lack of ventilation or drainage of the middle ear.

Procedure

General endotracheal anesthesia is given before adenoidectomy. A mouth gag is placed, and the soft and hard palate are assessed for evidence of a submucous cleft (Figure 4). A catheter is placed to retract the palate to assess the adenoid pad. Curettes of various sizes are then used to remove the adenoid tissue, taking care to avoid the ET orifices. Pressure and suction cautery are used to obtain hemostasis of the adenoid bed. Postoperative recovery is usually uneventful; some mild referred otalgia may occur.

Potential complications of adenoidectomy include postoperative hemorrhage, velopharyngeal incompetence, and anesthesia-related complications. Postoperative hemorrhage is rare (approximately 0.4%). Permanent velopharyngeal incompetence is rare unless there is an undiagnosed submucous cleft. Temporary changes in speech (increased nasality) may occur postoperatively, but resolve quickly.

References

1. Jyväkorpi M: A comparison of topical Emla cream with Bonain's solution for anesthesia of the tympanic membrane during tympanocentesis. *Eur Arch Otorhinolaryngol* 1996;253: 234-236.

2. Stool SE, Berg AO, Carney CT, et al: *Otitis Media With Effusion in Young Children*. Rockville, MD, Agency for Health Care Policy and Research, Public Health Services, U.S. Department of Health and Human Services, 1994. Clinical Practice Guideline No. 12, AHCPR Publication No. 94-0622.

3. Hsu GS, Levine SC, Giebink GS: Management of otitis media using Agency for Health Care Policy and Research guidelines. The Agency for Health Care Policy and Research. *Otolaryngol Head Neck Surg* 1998;118:437-443.

4. Rosenfeld RM, Goldsmith AJ, Tetlus L, et al: Quality of life for children with otitis media. *Arch Otolaryngol Head Neck Surg* 1997;123:1049-1054.

5. Hart MC, Nichols DS, Butler EM, et al: Childhood imbalance and chronic otitis media with effusion: effect of tympanostomy tube insertion on standardized tests of balance and locomotion. *Laryngoscope* 1998;108:665-670.

6. Oluwole M, Mills RP: Methods of selection for adenoidectomy in childhood otitis media with effusion. *Int J Pediatr Otorhinolaryngol* 1995;32:129-135.

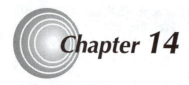

Chapter 14

Mastoiditis

B efore the 1940s, acute mastoiditis was the most common complication related to acute otitis media (AOM). With the development of antibiotics, the rate of acute mastoiditis has decreased from up to 50% in the 1930s to significantly less than 1%.[1] Some researchers have suggested that the incidence of acute mastoiditis may now be increasing, possibly related to attempts to decrease antibiotic use in response to rising bacterial resistance.

Mastoiditis is most common in young children without a significant medical history. Acute mastoiditis is an infectious continuum of AOM, just as the mastoid air cells are an anatomic continuum of the middle ear space. It is a disease spectrum that ranges from inflammation of the mastoid mucosa with periosteitis, to osteitis and actual bony destruction (coalescence) of the mastoid air cells. Clinical differentiation among the different stages of mastoiditis is important in choosing appropriate therapy (Table 1).

Anatomy and Pathophysiology

Understanding the spectrum and development of mastoiditis requires an understanding of the anatomy and pathophysiology of the mastoid air cell system. The middle ear space is connected to the mastoid cavity via the aditus ad antrum. The entire system is lined contiguously with mucosa. Thus, an infectious process involving the middle ear can easily travel through the antrum into the mastoid

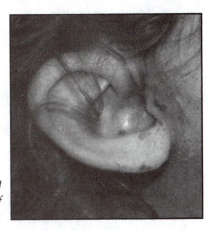

Figure 1: Clinical presentation of mastoiditis.

air cells. Studies have demonstrated the presence of mastoid inflammation from the first day of an acute middle ear infection. Although often described as tympanomastoiditis, this term has little clinical significance. The inflammation and edema of the mastoid air cell mucosa in tympanomastoiditis is readily reversible with treatment and resolution of AOM.

When the treatment and resolution of middle ear infection are delayed, the antrum (connection between the middle ear and mastoid) becomes obstructed with significant mucosal edema and eventually with granulation tissue. When this occurs, the mastoid cavity loses its drainage system, isolating it from the middle ear. If the infection is not treated expediently, the antral obstruction will become less reversible as granulation tissue and even osteogenesis develop. The isolated infection within the mastoid cavity eventually results in periosteitis of the air cells. Clinical findings include postauricular erythema and edema but no evidence of bony coalescence. At this stage, aggressive intravenous antibiotic therapy may still reverse the process.

Bony resorption and coalescence result when the periosteitis progresses to osteitis and pressure results in

Table 1: Clinical Spectrum of Mastoiditis

Acute otitis media

Acute tympanomastoiditis

Mastoiditis with periosteitis

Coalescent mastoiditis

Extension

- subperiosteal abscess
- petrositis
- Bezold's abscess
- intracranial complications

purulence. Coalescent mastoiditis requires surgical extirpation (mastoidectomy) to drain the abscess, as well as myringotomy tube placement to reestablish ventilation.

When coalescent mastoiditis is not appropriately treated, the purulence under pressure may erode and extend in several different directions, resulting in secondary complications. A subperiosteal abscess may occur with lateral extension, while petrositis, labyrinthitis, or facial nerve paralysis may occur with medial spread. Intracranial complications occur with superior and medial extension. Inferior penetration results in a Bezold's abscess if there is rupture through the mastoid tip, with a resultant posterior triangle neck abscess. Before the advent of antibiotics, subperiosteal abscesses occurred in approximately 20% of cases of coalescent mastoiditis, increasing to almost 50% of patients in the postantibiotic era.[1]

Clinical Presentation and Clinical Variants

The clinical presentation of mastoiditis in children varies, depending on the stage of infection. Clinical differentiation between acute mastoiditis with periosteitis versus coalescence is difficult without radiographic evaluation. The classic presentation is an acutely ill child with a protruding ear secondary to postauricular erythema and swelling (Figure 1). The symptom progression is fairly rapid, and is generally preceded by AOM. In a recent review, the most common predecessors were pain and fever lasting more than 4 days.[2] A review by Gliklich et al found that although pain was the most common presenting symptom, 45% of patients had no history of AOM.[3] This study indicated that the most common physical findings were an abnormal-appearing tympanic membrane (88%), fever (83%), a narrowed external auditory canal (80%), and postauricular edema (76%).

The availability of antibiotics for the treatment of AOM has dramatically decreased the incidence of mastoiditis. However, antibiotics have also created an entity referred to as *subacute* or *masked* mastoiditis. In this process, antibiotics only partially eradicate the mastoid infection, resulting in a subclinical infection. Whether the infection is secondary to inappropriate dosing, duration, or the type of antibiotic used, is unknown. The infection generally evolves insidiously, and patients often present with subtle, atypical findings. This delays clinical recognition of mastoiditis. A secondary complication, such as facial nerve paralysis, meningitis, or epidural abscess, may be the first indicator of mastoid disease. A high level of suspicion is therefore necessary for an expeditious diagnosis.

Chronic mastoiditis is synonymous with chronic suppurative otitis media (CSOM), and is addressed at length in Chapter 12. In chronic mastoiditis, the tympanic membrane is perforated, with long-standing otorrhea and chronic inflammation of the middle ear and mastoid cavity. This process evolves slowly, often requiring a tympanomastoidectomy.

Microbiology

A mixed flora, including gram-positive, gram-negative, and anaerobic organisms, may be cultured from patients with mastoiditis. The most commonly cultured organisms in acute disease include *Streptococcus pneumoniae*, *Haemophilus influenzae*, and *Staphylococcus aureus*. These are common in AOM as well. Gram-negative bacilli, such as *Proteus*, *Escherichia coli*, and *Pseudomonas*, may also be cultured, although they are more common in masked and chronic mastoiditis (CSOM). Anaerobic organisms have been cultured in up to 80% of patients undergoing mastoid surgery.[4]

Many other disease processes may present or masquerade as mastoiditis. Because of the prevalence and similarities in presentation, neoplastic disorders may go initially undiagnosed. Malignancies presenting as mastoiditis include rhabdomyosarcoma, histiocytosis X, leukemia, and T-cell lymphoma. Langerhans' cell histiocytosis (previously referred to as eosinophilic granuloma), Hand-Schüller-Christian disease, and Letterer-Siwe disease may all present as chronic otitis media (OM), often with a mass within the external auditory canal and lytic lesions on radiograph. Treatment ranges from surgical curettage and low-dose radiation to intensive chemotherapy.

Unusual infectious etiologies presenting with mastoiditis include atypical mycobacterial disease, tuberculosis, and fungal infection, particularly that caused by *Aspergillus fumigatus*. Autoimmune diseases, such as Wegener's granulomatosis, have also been described.

Radiology

Radiographic imaging is important in the differentiation between acute mastoiditis with and without coalescence. Temporal bone computed tomography (CT) defines the bony architecture of the middle ear and mastoid air cells and delineates the stage of the inflammatory process. Clouding of the mastoid air cells and middle ear is the earliest finding in mastoiditis. The bony air cells remain intact. With progression of the infectious process, the bony trabeculae become ill defined, eventually progressing to coalescence.

Treatment

The treatment of mastoiditis may be either medical or medical-surgical, depending on the stage at diagnosis. Early mastoiditis without evidence of coalescence, ie, only periosteitis, can be treated with intravenous antibiotic therapy alone. Empiric coverage with a third-generation cephalosporin, such as cefotaxime (Claforan®) or ceftriaxone (Rocephin®), is usually adequate. A tympanocentesis or myringotomy is performed to obtain culture information and to facilitate drainage and ventilation. Intravenous antibiotics are continued for 48 to 72 hours until a clinical response is demonstrated, followed by a 2- to 3-week course of outpatient oral antibiotics. A retrospective study examining early intravenous antibiotic therapy, wide myringotomy, and aspiration of any subperiosteal abscess demonstrated a decreased need for cortical mastoidectomy and reduced hospitalization time.[5]

Surgical therapy is required for patients with evidence of coalescence, nonresponsiveness to antibiotics, or secondary complications (Table 2). Mastoidectomy allows for drainage of the loculated mastoid abscess and reinstates ventilation (antrostomy). Most otolaryngologists perform a cortical mastoidectomy with opening of the aditus ad antrum. Great effort should be made to open the obstructed antrum, which provides drainage and ventilation. A tympanostomy tube should be placed, although an extremely edematous external canal may make this procedure difficult. An elevated white blood cell count, ptosis of the auricle, and fever on admission may be risk factors for surgical intervention.[3]

Harley et al found that in the absence of a subperiosteal abscess or other complications, there was no significant

---

Table 2: Indications for Mastoidectomy

- Coalescent mastoiditis
- Unresponsiveness to conventional antibiotics
- Secondary complications

---

difference between children treated with intravenous antibiotics and myringotomies versus those with mastoidectomies.[2] On the other hand, most clinicians believe that evidence of coalescence requires mastoidectomy. Although mastoidectomy is usually performed as soon as coalescent mastoiditis is diagnosed, intracranial complications may delay surgery until the patient is stabilized from the life-threatening situation.

References

1.   Spiegel JH, Lustig LR, Lee KC, et al: Contemporary presentation and management of a spectrum of mastoid abscesses. *Laryngoscope* 1998;108:822-828.

2.   Harley EH, Sdralis T, Berkowitz RG: Acute mastoiditis in children: a 12-year retrospective study. *Otolaryngol Head Neck Surg* 1997;116:26-30.

3.   Gliklich RE, Eavey RD, Iannuzzi RA, et al: A contemporary analysis of acute mastoiditis. *Arch Otolaryngol Head Neck Surg* 1996;122:135-139.

4.   Maharaj D, Jadwat A, Fernandes CM, et al: Bacteriology in acute mastoiditis. *Arch Otolaryngol Head Neck Surg* 1987;113: 514-515.

5.   Khafif A, Halperin D, Hochman I, et al: Acute mastoiditis: a 10-year review. *Am J Otolaryngol* 1998;19:170-173.

Selected Readings

Danino J, Joachims HZ, Ben-Arieh Y, et al: T cell lymphoma of the ear presenting as mastoiditis. *J Laryngol Otol* 1997;111: 852-854.

Grewal DS, Bhargava P, Mistry B, et al: Tuberculoma of the mastoid. *J Laryngol Otol* 1995;109:232-235.

Holt GR, Gates GA: Masked mastoiditis. *Laryngoscope* 1983; 93:1034-1037.

Nadol JB Jr, Eavey RD: Acute and chronic mastoiditis: clinical presentation, diagnosis, and management. *Curr Clin Top Infect Dis* 1995;15:204-229.

Moussa AE, Abou-Elhmd KA: Wegener's granulomatosis presenting as mastoiditis. *Ann Otol Rhinol Laryngol* 1998;107:560-563.

Shaida A, Siddiqui N: Imaging quiz case 2. Tuberculous mastoiditis causing a facial palsy. *Arch Otolaryngol Head Neck Surg* 1998;124:341, 343.

Stewart MG, Troendle-Atkins J, Starke JR, et al: Nontuberculous mycobacterial mastoiditis. *Arch Otolaryngol Head Neck Surg* 1995;121:225-228.

Yates PD, Upile T, Axon PR, et al: *Aspergillus* mastoiditis in a patient with acquired immunodeficiency syndrome. *J Laryngol Otol* 1997;111:560-561.

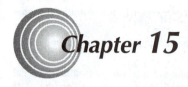

Chapter 15

Cholesteatoma

C holesteatoma is an epithelium-lined mass that may occur within the external auditory canal, middle ear, and mastoid.[1,2] Cholesteatoma is a misnomer; it contains neither fat nor cholesterol. Because cholesteatoma is essentially skin that is growing in an incorrect place, a more appropriate name might be keratoma.

Cholesteatomas are classified as either congenital or acquired; each is equally destructive if not appropriately identified and treated. The result of these keratinizing stratified squamous epithelial tumors is an accumulation of desquamated epithelium that expands and destroys over time. The bone erosion and resulting sequelae result from both mass effect and enzymatic activity. Aural (ear) cholesteatomas are defined by their presence medial to the normal position of the tympanic membrane, and are composed of all the skin layers.

Many consider pediatric cholesteatomas to be more 'aggressive' than those occurring in adults. This is evident at the time of surgery, as children commonly manifest more extensive disease. The rate of recurrence is also higher in children than in adults.

Pathogenesis

The destructive properties of cholesteatoma, including the bony erosion, result from the expanding mass and the enzymatic production of the epithelium. The destructive pathway of the mass depends on the area of initial epithelial invasion and the mucosal folds and ligaments that

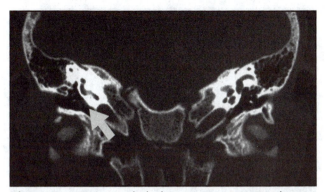

Figure 1-a: *Congenital cholesteatoma. CT scan demonstrating middle ear cholesteatoma. Used with permission from Handler S, Myer C: Ear, Nose, and Throat Disease in Children. Hamilton, Ontario, BC Decker, 1998.*

'guide' it. When the epitympanum is the epicenter, the cholesteatoma extends into the antrum, mastoid, or inferiorly into the middle ear. A cholesteatoma initially invading through a posterosuperior perforation may first extend into the mesotympanum, then posteriorly into the mastoid. Eventually, extensive cholesteatomas unrelated to the epicenter result in large invasive masses occupying the entire middle ear and mastoid. Ossicular erosion is common with extensive cholesteatoma, while labyrinthine, fallopian canal, and tegmen erosion occur in later-stage cholesteatomas.

The bony destruction results from both mass effect and enzymatic activity. The bony resorption that occurs as the cholesteatoma expands may result in an 'automastoidectomy'. The squamous epithelium has also been shown to produce enzymes (collagenases) whose activity intensifies during an active infection. These collagenases are produced at the epithelial and subepithelial junction. Granulation tissue results from infection, and its enzymatic production and activity are enhanced during infection.

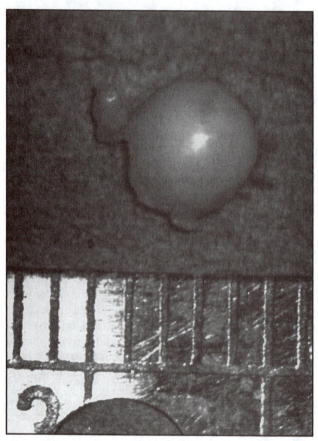

Figure 1-b: *Surgical specimen of a cholesteatoma 'pearl.'* Used with permission from Handler S, Myer C: Ear, Nose, and Throat Disease in Children. *Hamilton, Ontario, BC Decker, 1998.*

An infected cholesteatoma is an excellent culture medium for both aerobic and anaerobic organisms, most commonly *Pseudomonas aeruginosa* and *Proteus*. When medi-

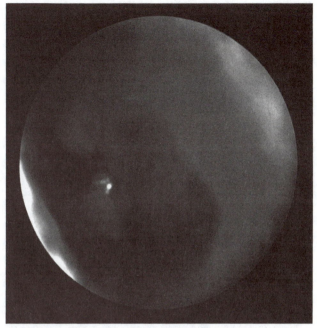

Figure 1-c: Clinical photograph demonstrating congenital cholesteatoma pearl in the anterior two thirds of the tympanic membrane.

cally treating an infected cholesteatoma, adequate gram-negative bacteria coverage is imperative.

Congenital Cholesteatoma

Aural cholesteatomas may be classified as either congenital or acquired. Congenital cholesteatomas may occur in the middle ear, external auditory canal, mastoid, petrous apex, or cerebellopontile angle. Researchers believe they occur secondary to displaced epithelial rests present at birth. Congenital middle ear cholesteatomas do not generally present until 5 years of age, unless identi-

Table 1: Sade Staging for the Atelectatic Tympanic Membrane

Stage 1	Slightly retracted
Stage 2	Draped over incus
Stage 3	Draped over promontory
Stage 4	Adhesive tympanic membrane (over promontory)
Stage 5	Tympanic membrane adhesive and perforated

fied earlier by an astute clinician viewing an asymptomatic whitish 'pearl' behind an intact tympanic membrane. Two thirds of these masses present in the anterior superior quadrant, although they may occur in other quadrants (Figure 1, a-c). To be considered 'congenital', there should be no history of otitis media (OM), otorrhea, or otologic surgery, including placement of tympanostomy tubes.

Because OM is relatively common in the pediatric population, the diagnosis of congenital cholesteatoma is often delayed. In addition, differentiation between acquired and congenital disease may be difficult.

Acquired Cholesteatoma

The two types of acquired cholesteatomas are primary and secondary. Each generally results from OM and eustachian tube dysfunction. Primary acquired cholesteatomas, also referred to as attic cholesteatomas, result from invagination of the tympanic membrane. This occurs when eustachian tube dysfunction causes chronic negative pressure, which can be as great as -600 cm H_2O (Figure 2). Secondary acquired cholesteatomas generally result from ingrowth of squamous epithelium through the margins of a chronic tympanic membrane perforation.

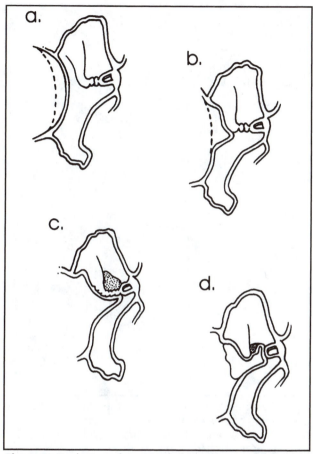

Figure 2: *Evolution of acquired cholesteatoma secondary to chronic negative middle ear pressure. Adapted from Bluestone CD, Klein JO, eds:* Otitis Media in Infants and Children, *2nd ed. Philadelphia, WB Saunders, 1995.*

Researchers believe a primary acquired cholesteatoma results from prolonged negative pressure and eustachian tube dysfunction. The chronic negative pressure and re-

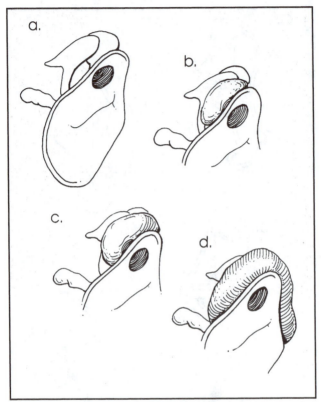

Figure 3: Evolution of tympanic membrane retraction pocket into cholesteatoma. Adapted from Bluestone CD, Klein JO, eds: Otitis Media in Infants and Children, 2nd ed. Philadelphia, WB Saunders, 1995.

traction results in a flaccid and atelectatic tympanic membrane. The pars flaccida, the most 'flaccid' area of the tympanic membrane, becomes a localized retraction pocket. As this pocket reaches a critical depth, failure to clear trapped desquamated epithelium results in formation of a cholesteatoma (Figure 3). This may occur in the

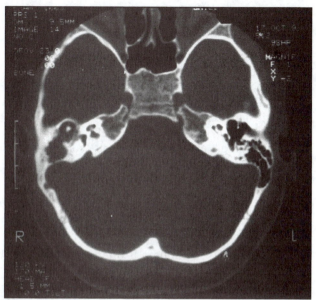

Figure 4: *CT scan demonstrating cholesteatoma of the temporal bone.*

pars flaccida as well as the posterior superior aspect of the pars tensa (Figure 4). The Sade method of classifying pars tensa retraction suggests grades from 1 to 5 (Table 1).

Primary acquired cholesteatoma is most common. A review of more than 1,000 adults and children with cholesteatoma demonstrated that the attic (epitympanum) was the most frequent location (42%), followed by the posterior-superior tympanic membrane (31%). Children with cleft palates who have a functional eustachian tube obstruction have an increased incidence of primary acquired cholesteatoma, which occurs in up to 7% of this population. This contrasts with the rare occurrence of cholesteatoma in the Eskimo population, where middle ear disease is related to a patulous eustachian tube rather than obstruction.

In secondary acquired cholesteatoma, the more unusual types result from squamous invasion into the middle ear through a chronic tympanic membrane perforation. Iatrogenic implantation of skin during surgery or, rarely, tympanostomy tube placement, may also result in secondarily acquired cholesteatoma. These cholesteatomas occur most frequently with marginal perforation, where the annulus is dehiscent and external canal epithelium may migrate into the middle ear. Theoretically, chronic infection of the middle ear mucosa prevents 'contact inhibition' and allows for epithelial migration into the middle ear cleft. Interestingly, only cholesteatoma and tympanic membrane epithelium demonstrate migratory ability, while oral, skin, and vocal cord epithelium do not.

Diagnosis

Early diagnosis in children is often difficult. Often subtle symptoms are likely to be missed until significant otologic destruction has occurred. Even with hearing loss, children rarely complain, especially if the loss is unilateral.

Pain is unusual unless it is a harbinger of an impending intracranial or intratemporal complication. Although foul otorrhea is common and easily identifiable, symptoms and signs that are difficult to relate, such as tinnitus, aural fullness, or even vertigo, often go unreported or even unrecognized. Obvious signs, however, such as severe vertigo, facial paralysis, nausea and vomiting, or change in consciousness, should alert the physician to the presence of cholesteatoma or chronic OM.

Otoscopy often reveals a large amount of discolored debris in the external ear canal or a crust overlying the epitympanum, which requires suctioning or removal before accurate identification of the cholesteatomatous epicenter. A shiny, white, flaky mass of keratin is seen erupting through the posterosuperior drum or epitympanum. The complete extent of the mass may not be fully appreciated because of temporal bone anatomy. Granulation tissue or polyps, often associated with the cholesteatoma and chronic inflammation, may impede adequate visualization. In an early congenital cholesteatoma, a small white 'pearl' is usually visualized anterosuperiorly behind an intact tympanic membrane.

Evaluation

A preoperative audiometric evaluation is imperative. Children most commonly have a conductive hearing loss, although some have normal or almost-normal hearing. Normal hearing occurs, despite ossicular erosion, when cholesteatoma acts as a conductor between the tympanic membrane and stapes or oval window. The risk of 'worsening' of hearing with surgery, especially in children with normal hearing, should be stressed. A sensorineural hearing loss is extremely important to identify preoperatively, as it may indicate a labyrinthine fistula or serous labyrinthitis. Once again, although tympanometry usually demonstrates increased impedance, it may also be normal.

Temporal bone computed tomography (CT) may be quite helpful in demonstrating the extent of the cholesteatoma, as well as the status of the ossicles, labyrinth, tegmen, and fallopian canal. Many otologic surgeons obtain a CT preoperatively. Plain films and magnetic resonance imaging (MRI) have limited use. MRI may aid in the diagnosis of intracranial complications.

Intervention

Surgery is the management for aural cholesteatoma. The only role of medical management is in the treatment of an infection preoperatively. Medical management involves both topical antibiotics with antipseudomonal activity as well as oral antibiotics. Ciprofloxacin (Cipro®) has excellent antipseudomonal activity, but its oral form is not approved for the pediatric population. An actively draining ear may often be returned to a 'dry' state before surgery with aggressive medical treatment. Preoperative treatment of infection greatly aids the surgical procedure by decreasing middle ear edema and vascularity.

Prevention of cholesteatoma requires early identification of tympanic membrane changes and active attempts at reversal of retraction. Eustachian tube dysfunction must be directly addressed and bypassed. Retraction pockets, especially in the area of the epitympanum, require aggressive pressure equalization (ie, tympanostomy tubes) and vigilant monitoring. Occasionally, the placement of tympanostomy tubes reverses the early tympanic membrane retraction. When the retraction pocket is more 'end-stage' and the atelectatic drum is more adhesive, intraoperative injection of saline may occasionally allow for 'eversion' of the pocket. If the retraction pocket cannot be everted and the 'deep' portion of the pocket cannot be visualized, definitive otologic surgery is necessary.

The two goals of cholesteatoma surgery are to provide a 'safe' ear and to restore function (hearing). A safe ear is one in which all disease has been eradicated. There is no role for a 'debulking' procedure. If there is any question of residual disease at the end of the procedure, a 'second-look' operation or a canal wall-down procedure should be performed. Cholesteatoma surgery requires both an in-depth understanding of the otologic anatomy and an understanding of the recidivism and aggressiveness of this disease.

The surgical approach to cholesteatoma depends on the site and extent of the disease, and the patient's health and reliability in returning for follow-up. In the rare instance of an early cholesteatoma that is limited to the middle ear, the entire disease may be removed through a middle ear exploration. Generally, however, both middle ear and mastoid surgery is necessary.

A mastoidectomy entails surgical exposure and removal of the mastoid air cells, as well as opening the aditus ad antrum. A mastoidectomy allows for removal of the dis-

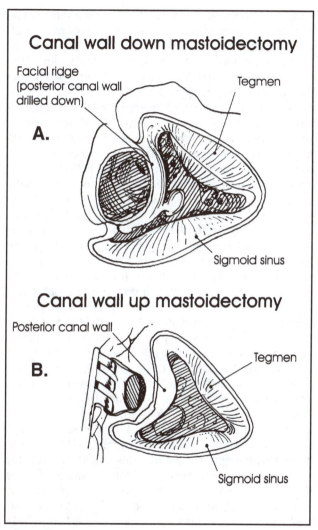

Figure 5: (a) Canal wall-down mastoidectomy with the posterior canal wall drilled down. (b) Canal wall-up mastoidectomy with an intact posterior canal wall.

ease and formation of an opening between the mastoid and middle ear that, in certain approaches, provides a direct connection between the external auditory canal and the mastoid cavity (canal wall-down mastoidectomy). The extent of mastoid and middle ear involvement determines the most appropriate approach.

A mastoidectomy may be categorized as either the canal wall-up (CWU) mastoidectomy/'closed' technique or the canal wall-down (CWD) mastoidectomy/'open' technique.[3,4] The optimal choice depends on whether the posterior external canal wall is maintained (CWU) or if the posterior canal is drilled down, allowing for direct visualization and access to the mastoid bowl (CWD) (Figure 5, a-b). The 'exteriorized ear' with the CWD approach allows the surgeon to directly visualize and remove any recurrent cholesteatoma within the mastoid cavity. A significant disadvantage is the nonphysiologic nature of a mastoid bowl, which lacks the self-cleaning mechanism of the external canal, resulting in lifelong outpatient débridement and an increased difficulty of ossicular reconstruction. In contrast, the CWU mastoidectomy maintains the external auditory canal with its self-cleaning mechanism, but at the cost of potentially remaining occult cholesteatoma. In the CWU mastoidectomy, a 'second-look' exploration may be required 6 months after the initial procedure to rule out occult disease. Recently, otoendoscopes have been discussed as a possible replacement for selected 'second-look' procedures.[5] Although researchers have long believed that the CWD mastoidectomy results in poorer hearing, this assumption is being questioned. A recent study examining sound transmission through the middle ear in CWU and CWD mastoidectomy demonstrated that CWD mastoidectomy causes less than 10-dB changes in sound transmission relative to the CWU, as long as the middle ear air space is aerated.[3]

The goals of surgery are primarily to eradicate keratinizing squamous epithelium from the temporal bone and, secondarily, to preserve or restore hearing. Continued follow-up by an otolaryngologist is essential to prevent and control recurrent disease.

Debate is ongoing about whether CWU or CWD mastoidectomy is the more appropriate management of pediatric cholesteatoma. Those who favor CWD mastoidectomy cite the aggressiveness and unsatisfactory control of this disease in children. Those who favor CWU mastoidectomy cite the difficulty in managing the mastoid cavity. The literature also supports the favorable results with the use of CWU mastoidectomy for pediatric cholesteatoma.[4] CWU mastoidectomy supporters suggest that the trade-off of a planned second-stage surgery, with its minimal morbidity, is well worth the long-term results of an ear with useful hearing without the need for chronic medical care. Considering these variables, most otolaryngologists individualize their approach to pediatric cholesteatoma.

Complications and Sequelae of Cholesteatoma and Cholesteatoma Surgery

The most common sequela of a cholesteatoma is hearing loss up to 50 dB secondary to ossicular erosion. A labyrinthine fistula may be present in up to 10% of patients with vertigo and sensorineural hearing loss. Both an acutely infected cholesteatoma and a chronically expanding cholesteatoma may result in a facial nerve paralysis. Treatment of facial nerve paralysis includes cholesteatoma removal with facial nerve decompression, without opening the nerve sheath. An encephalocele or brain herniation may occur when tegmen dehiscence results from either cholesteatoma erosion or iatrogenic drilling of the tegmen.

The complications resulting from cholesteatoma surgery are very similar to those that may result from an untreated cholesteatoma. Complications of acute otitis media may also occur secondary to cholesteatoma. Meningitis secondary to tegmen erosion, abscesses (subdural, epidural, or brain), sigmoid sinus thrombosis, and subperiosteal abscess are all potential sequelae, and are reviewed in Chapter 16.

References

1.   Michaels L: Biology of cholesteatoma. *Otolaryngol Clin North Am* 1989;22:869-881.

2.   Sie KC: Cholesteatoma in children. *Pediatr Clin North Am* 1996;43:1245-52.

3.   Whittemore KR Jr, Merchant SN, Rosowski JJ: Acoustic mechanisms: canal wall-up versus canal wall-down mastoidectomy. *Otolaryngol Head Neck Surg* 1998;118:751-761.

4.   Dodson EE, Hashisaki GT, Hobgood TC, et al: Intact canal wall mastoidectomy with tympanoplasty for cholesteatoma in children. *Laryngoscope* 1998;108:977-983.

5.   Rosenberg SI, Silverstein H, Hoffer M, et al: Use of endoscopes for chronic ear surgery in children. *Arch Otolaryngol Head Neck Surg* 1995;121:870-872.

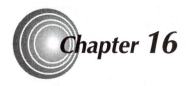

Chapter 16

Complications of Otitis Media

C omplications secondary to otitis media (OM) have decreased drastically since the advent of antibiotics. Otitis media-related intracranial complications, for example, have been reduced from approximately 2.3% of cases during the preantibiotic era, to the current rate of 0.04% to 0.15%. Despite the use of appropriate antimicrobial therapy, however, complications occur when infection spreads beyond the confines of the temporal bone. These often result from subacute or chronic ear infections.

Complications are classified as either intratemporal or intracranial (Table 1). Intratemporal complications include mastoiditis, petrositis, labyrinthitis, and facial nerve paralysis. Cholesteatoma, retraction pockets, and ossicular erosion may also be considered intratemporal complications and have been reviewed in previous chapters. Intracranial complications include sigmoid sinus thrombophlebitis, brain abscess, otitic hydrocephalus, meningitis, and subdural abscess (Figure 1).

Complications of OM often are related to subacute and chronic infections. Diagnosis of an impending complication requires a high index of suspicion. An acute otitis media (AOM) that persists for more than 2 weeks or that recurs within 3 weeks may be considered a precursor to a complication. Fetid discharge within the ear canal in conjunction with an acute infection indicates anaerobic or-

Table 1: Complications of Otitis Media

Intratemporal

- Mastoiditis
- Petrositis
- Labyrinthitis
- Facial nerve paralysis

Intracranial

- Sigmoid sinus thrombophlebitis
- Brain abscess
- Otitic hydrocephalus
- Meningitis
- Subdural abscess

ganisms, and may be associated with an impending complication. Signs and symptoms of complications include fever associated with chronic perforation, edema of the posterosuperior canal wall skin, a pinna displaced inferolaterally (mastoiditis), or retro-orbital pain on the side of the infected ear (petrositis).

Certain signs and symptoms should be considered emergencies when found in conjunction with an acute or chronic OM. Facial nerve paralysis in conjunction with an OM requires immediate attention. The decision to perform a myringotomy or mastoidectomy depends on whether the infection is related to an acute OM or a chronic OM with or without cholesteatoma. Acute vertigo and decreased hearing in a child with OM requires immediate attention because of the potential for suppurative labyrinthitis. This diagnosis requires immediate hospitalization and intravenous antibiotics. A change of mental status or coma in conjunction with OM may indicate meningitis, otitic hy-

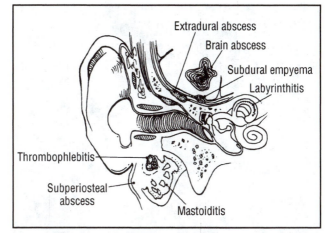

Figure 1: *Intratemporal complications include mastoiditis, petrositis, labyrinthitis, and facial nerve paralysis. Intracranial complications include sigmoid thrombophlebitis, brain abscess, otitic hydrocephalus, meningitis, and subdural abscess. Adapted from Bluestone CD, Klein JO, eds:* Otitis Media in Infants and Children, *2nd ed. Philadelphia, WB Saunders, 1995.*

drocephalus, or subdural or brain abscess. Focal neurologic deficits, such as seizures, alert the physician to an intracranial complication.

Mastoiditis

The mastoid cavity is the anatomic extension of the middle ear space; acute mastoiditis is the natural pathologic extension of AOM. An AOM often results in concomitant inflammation of mastoid air cells without osteitis. The process is reversed with the resolution of the OM. If resolution does not occur, a subacute stage, often referred to as 'masked mastoiditis,' ensues. In masked mastoiditis, the signs and symptoms are similar to an AOM but are persistent, and the inflammation continues with-

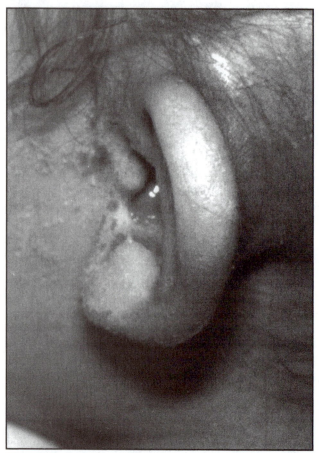

Figure 2: *Patients with acute coalescent mastoiditis present with erythema and edema over the mastoid and an inferiorly displaced, protruding pinna.*

out evidence of osteitis or bony destruction. Tympanocentesis is both diagnostic and therapeutic, identifying the causative organism and promoting drainage. Masked mastoiditis often responds to the appropriate antibiotic.

An acute coalescent mastoiditis results if the infection persists. The persistent infection causes bony destruction of the mastoid air cells and coalescence. Patients with acute coalescent mastoiditis present with erythema and edema over the mastoid and an inferiorly displaced, protruding pinna (Figure 2). There may be postauricular fluctuance and skin breakdown, as well as an external canal swollen posterosuperiorly and filled with debris. The children are often acutely ill, with fevers and other signs of systemic illness.

The purulence within the mastoid cavity can extend in many different directions, resulting in additional suppurative complications. Lateral spread of the exudate results in a subperiosteal abscess. Anterior spread into the neck below the pinna or sternocleidomastoid results in a Bezold's abscess. Petrositis occurs with medial spread into the petrous bone, and posterior spread may result in calvarial osteomyelitis.

Computed tomography (CT) is often critical to the diagnosis of acute coalescent mastoiditis. CT aids in the differentiation of early mastoiditis without osteitis, which responds to parenteral antibiotics, and coalescent mastoiditis, which requires both antimicrobial and surgical therapy (Figure 3). CT may also help diagnose other complications.

Treatment of acute coalescent mastoiditis hinges on appropriate antimicrobial therapy and adequate drainage (mastoidectomy). Uncomplicated coalescent mastoiditis most often results from *Streptococcus pneumoniae* or *Haemophilus influenzae*. An intravenous antibiotic, usually a third-generation cephalosporin, which is active against β-lactamase-producing organisms, is most appropriate. Drainage is provided by a cortical mastoidectomy. This allows for exoneration of the mastoid air cells, removal of obstructing granulation tissue, and culture identification of the organism(s).

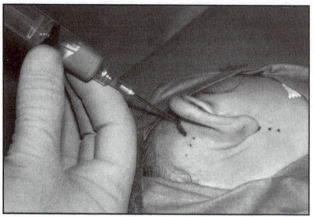

Figure 3: *Lateral spread of the mastoiditis results in a subperiosteal abscess.*

Labyrinthitis

Labyrinthitis related to otitis media occurs most often from infectious spread through the round or oval window, or through a congenital defect of the inner ear. Labyrinthitis results either from spread of the actual bacteria, as in suppurative labyrinthitis, or from spread of the bacterial toxin, as in serous labyrinthitis. Suppurative labyrinthitis is rare and potentially life threatening, resulting in extreme toxicity, severe vertigo, and often permanent sensorineural hearing loss. Suppurative infections may, in turn, seed the cerebrospinal fluid or meninges, resulting in intracranial complications. Treatment includes parenteral antibiotics and surgical therapy if there is associated cholesteatoma or chronic OM.

Serous labyrinthitis results from cochlear and vestibular irritation secondary to the spread of bacterial toxins. The clinical presentation and sequelae are less severe than suppurative labyrinthitis; the mixed hearing loss is usually reversible and the vertigo is less severe. Treatment

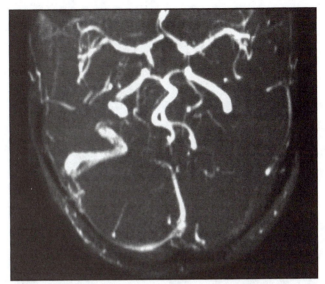

Figure 4: *Magnetic resonance angiography provides increased information on the status of sinus flow. This demonstrates absent flow of left transverse and sigmoid sinus.*

includes culture-directed antimicrobial therapy, supportive care, and possibly corticosteroids to decrease the inflammatory response.

Facial Paralysis

Facial paralysis may result from either an AOM or a coalescent mastoiditis. The facial nerve courses through the middle ear and mastoid. Congenital bony dehiscence may occur in up to 50% of the population. The facial nerve may be quite vulnerable to middle ear pathology. An AOM in the presence of a dehiscent facial nerve may result in facial paralysis secondary to the toxic effects on the exposed nerve. Facial paralysis secondary to mastoiditis or cholesteatoma results from bony erosion, nerve compression, and vascular occlusion.

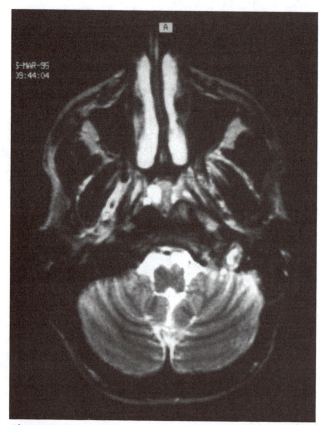

Figure 5: T2 MRI demonstrating thrombosis in left jugular canal.

The significant facial tone in children may make the diagnosis of facial nerve paralysis difficult. A CT is required to determine if the paralysis is secondary to an acute OM or chronic OM to select appropriate treatment.

Facial nerve paralysis related to AOM is expected to resolve within 24 hours after myringotomy tube placement and appropriate antimicrobial therapy. If resolution does not occur, surgical decompression should be considered. In contrast, facial nerve paralysis secondary to chronic OM requires surgical therapy, mastoidectomy with or without facial nerve decompression, and antimicrobial therapy.

Petrositis

The petrous apex is a poorly pneumatized area that may become inflamed and coalescent as a complication of OM. Secondary to its poor pneumatization, the osteitis generally begins with inflammation of the marrow spaces rather than the air cells (as in mastoiditis). The classic clinical triad, Gradenigo's syndrome, includes ipsilateral OM, severe retro-orbital pain, and ipsilateral lateral rectus palsy. CT with contrast demonstrates petrous apex coalescence (Figure 6, a-b). Treatment is surgical: myringotomy tube placement and drainage of the petrous apex. The petrous apex is determined by the pneumatization pattern most accessible to the area of coalescence. Appropriate antibiotic therapy is required as well.

Meningitis

Meningitis is the most common intracranial complication secondary to either acute or chronic OM. There are three routes of spread: hematogenous, the most common; direct spread, which is often through a dural or inner ear dehiscence; or local thrombophlebitis. Chronic OM, as opposed to AOM, most often results in meningitis from direct spread via a dural dehiscence or labyrinthine fistula.

Children present with classic signs of meningitis, including photophobia, headache, fever, and nuchal rigidity. Changes consistent with meningeal inflammation include Kernig's and Brudzinski's signs. A lumbar puncture (LP) should be performed to determine the causative organism, and the cerebrospinal fluid opening pressure and the protein, glucose, and white blood cell count

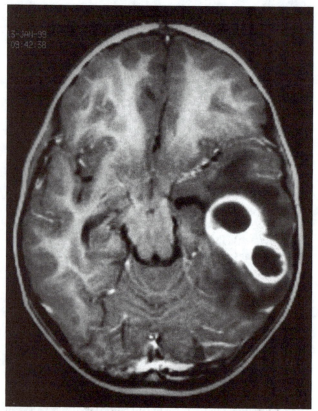

Figure 6a: *Head CT with contrast demonstrating large temporal lobe abscess after acute otitis media.*

should be determined. Intracranial imaging, usually a CT with contrast, should be obtained to rule out an intracranial mass that could precipitate cerebral herniation during an LP.

Culture-directed parenteral antibiotics are required to eradicate the infectious etiology. Parenteral corticosteroids that decrease cerebral inflammation have also been

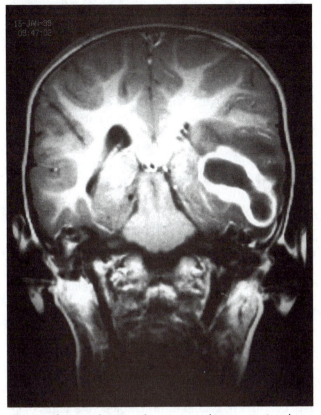

Figure 6b: *Head CT with contrast demonstrating large temporal lobe abscess after acute otitis media.*

recommended to decrease the risk of sensorineural hearing loss. Myringotomy with or without tube placement is performed on children with concomitant AOM. Children found to have either an abnormal connection between the middle ear and meninges, or a chronic OM with or without cholesteatoma, should undergo otologic surgery as soon as they can tolerate general anesthesia.

Sigmoid Sinus Thrombosis

Sigmoid sinus thrombosis or thrombophlebitis is a rare complication arising from inflammation in the mastoid air cells adjacent to the sigmoid sinus. The inflammation within the mastoid penetrates the adventitia and the wall of the sigmoid sinus, eventually resulting in thrombosis. The thrombus may become infected and enlarge. Subsequent embolization through the internal jugular vein may result in additional complications, such as empyema and joint infections.

Patients may be completely asymptomatic or severely ill. The classic presentation includes spiking fevers and chills secondary to intermittent bacteremia. There may be pain and edema over the mastoid secondary to occlusion of the mastoid emissary vein (Griesinger's sign). Other signs may include those of increased intracranial pressure, including headache, altered mental status, and seizures. Sigmoid sinus thrombophlebitis may produce intracranial complications such as cavernous sinus thrombosis, meningitis, or brain abscesses.

Identification of sigmoid sinus thrombosis demands a high level of suspicion. Magnetic resonance imaging (MRI) is considered the gold standard for diagnosis; a high signal demonstrated on both T1- and T2-weighted images is confirmatory. Magnetic resonance angiography provides increased information on the status of sinus flow (Figures 4 and 5). Routine CT, on the other hand, often misses sigmoid sinus thrombosis.

Management of sigmoid sinus thrombophlebitis includes appropriate antimicrobial therapy and surgery. The surgical treatment involves mastoidectomy with unroofing of the sigmoid sinus, drainage of any perisinuous abscesses, and removal of granulation tissue. The presence of a septic thrombus requires opening the sinus and removing the infected clot. Rarely, the internal jugular vein requires ligation to prevent embolization. The use of anticoagulants such as heparin, warfarin (Coumadin®), or urokinase remains controversial.

Otitic Hydrocephalus

Otitic hydrocephalus, ie, increased intracranial pressure without intracranial abnormalities, may occur secondary to AOM. The pathogenesis of otitic hydrocephalus is unknown, but is thought to be related to sigmoid sinus thrombosis. Researchers believe it results from decreased blood flow to the arachnoid granulation tissue, with a subsequent decrease in cerebrospinal fluid (CSF) absorption.

Children with otitic hydrocephalus present with evidence of increased intracranial pressure, such as papilledema, blurred vision, headaches, and vomiting. Papilledema may result in optic atrophy and subsequent blindness. This mandates that the patient undergo ongoing visual monitoring, including visual field testing. Diagnostic work-up includes a CT, which demonstrates normal-sized ventricles. LP is performed after ruling out intracranial masses. Opening CSF pressure may be as high as 300 mm H_2O with a normal protein and glucose content.

Treatment includes mastoidectomy to treat the sigmoid sinus thrombosis, and methods to decrease intracranial pressure. Management to decrease intracranial pressure includes repeated LPs, acetazolamide, and corticosteroids. Occasionally, placement of a lumboperitoneal shunt is necessary.

Brain Abscess

Otogenic brain abscesses may result from acute or chronic OM. Brain abscesses evolve in four clinical stages: invasion, localization, enlargement, and termination. Diagnosis may be difficult, depending on the clinical stage of the infection. Initially, a zone of encephalitis surrounds the abscess. Children often have low-grade fever and drowsiness. During localization, the abscess is 'quiescent' and the child is clinically asymptomatic for 2 to 3 weeks. Over 5 to 6 weeks, a fibrous capsule surrounds the abscess with gradual enlargement. During this stage there is a mass effect, with development of seizures and other localizing symptoms, depending on areas of involvement. Finally, the abscess results in either cerebral herniation or rupture into a ventricle or subarachnoid space. A rapid and often fatal outcome results.

Diagnosis may be made with a head CT scan with contrast or MRI (Figure 6, a-b). A ring-enhancing mass is characteristic within the brain parenchyma, most often within the temporal lobe or cerebellar regions. Depending on the stage, the abscess may not be readily apparent; repeated imaging several weeks later may be necessary. LP is contraindicated because of the risk of brain herniation.

Treatment includes appropriate antibiotic therapy to cover mixed flora, including both aerobic and anaerobic organisms. Intravenous prednisone may aid in decreasing surrounding brain edema. Surgical drainage of the abscess, through either a burr hole or craniotomy, should be performed as soon as the patient can tolerate general anesthesia. The underlying otologic disease should be treated as soon as the patient is stabilized.

Subdural Abscess

Subdural abscesses occur when purulence develops between the dura and arachnoid membrane. They occur more often secondary to sinusitis than to AOM. When associated with AOM, subdural abscess may develop as a result of direct extension or thrombophlebitis through venous channels.

On presentation, these children are extremely toxic from the mass effect and close proximity to the cerebral cortex. Focal neurologic findings such as seizures, decreased mental status, hemiplegia, and sensory deficits are common. Diagnosis may be made with contrast-enhanced CT or MRI.

Neurosurgical drainage of the subdural abscess should be performed through a burr hole or craniotomy. Appropriate long-term parenteral antibiotic therapy is necessary as well as, in certain circumstances, myringotomy. Formal otologic surgery is delayed until the patient is stabilized, after which the infectious breach may be explored.

It is important to remember that each complication may lead to a secondary complication if inadequately treated. The subsequent intracranial complications are more likely to extend medially than laterally. Inadequately treated mastoiditis may lead to facial paralysis or petrositis. Petrositis may produce additional intracranial suppuration, which may, in turn, lead to carotid artery rupture or facial paralysis. Ultimately, each complication may be fatal if inadequately treated.

Conclusion

A decrease in OM-related complications requires physicians to increase their level of suspicion for these events, particularly in children with prolonged infection. Failing to appropriately identify and treat these children may result in significant morbidity and even mortality.

Suggested Reading

Nissen AJ, Bui H: Complications of chronic otitis media. *Ear Nose Throat J* 1996;75:284-292.

Neely JG: Surgery of acute infections and their complications. In: Brackmann DE, ed. *Otologic Surgery*. Philadelphia, WB Saunders, 1994, pp 201-210.

Neely JG: Intratemporal and intracranial complications of otitis media. In: Bailey BJ, ed. *Head and Neck Surgery—Otolaryngology*. Philadelphia, JB Lippincott, 1993, pp 1607-1622.

Index

A

trimethoprim/sulfamethoxazole (TMP/SMX) (Bactrim™, Septra®) 51, 55, 83, 88, 89, 92, 94, 98, 100-102, 114, 146, 148, 156, 158, 161, 162, 173
tuberculosis 208
tumors 212
tuning fork tests 177
Turner's syndrome 145, 157
tymp-tap 195
tympanic membrane (TM) 9, 25, 26, 30, 31, 36, 62, 64, 67, 70-74, 76, 113, 120, 122, 123, 176, 183-185, 187, 194, 196, 198-200, 207, 212, 215, 216, 218, 219, 221, 222
tympanocentesis 50, 58, 61-63, 88, 103, 113, 144, 193-196, 209, 230
tympanogram 74, 76, 77, 85, 87, 129, 163, 176, 198
tympanomastoid surgery 189
tympanomastoidectomy 207
tympanomastoiditis 205, 206
tympanometry 10, 43, 77, 87, 172, 173, 176, 221
tympanoplasty 138, 185-187, 191
tympanosclerosis 72, 73, 78, 180

tympanostomy tube (TT) 37, 68, 87, 120, 121, 123, 126, 134, 136-138, 146, 148, 150, 156, 165-167, 180, 183, 185, 190, 193, 196-202, 209, 216, 220, 222

U

unconditioned responses 80
upper respiratory infection 61, 149
upper respiratory tract infections 14, 17, 28, 157, 158, 161
urokinase 239

V

vaccines 117, 153, 164, 165
Valsalva's maneuver 28, 29, 131, 163
Vancenase® 128
vancomycin 55
Vantin® 50, 83, 86, 102
varicella 128, 180
vascular disease 188
vasoconstrictors 131
ventilating tubes 19, 21, 37, 85, 129, 172, 185
ventilation 79, 131
vertigo 9, 220, 225, 228, 232
viral infection 10, 13, 16-22, 35, 49, 59-61, 114, 149, 153, 154, 157, 158, 161

vomiting 9, 93, 108, 109, 220, 239

W

Waldeyer's ring 201
warfarin (Coumadin®) 239
Wegener's granulomatosis 208
weight loss 34
withholding therapy 87, 105, 112, 115
Wymox® 88

X

xylitol sugar 148, 150, 156, 162, 163

Y

yawning 131

Z

Zithromax® 49, 83, 87, 102, 112